WEST OF ENGLAND EMERGENCY SERVICE VEHICLES

Dave Boulter

AMBERLEY

Front cover (upper): 12 April 2016 saw a police incident result in the full closure of Bristol's busy A432 Fishponds Road.

Front cover (lower): On 22 March 2010, on a very wet and windy Plymouth Hoe, six new aerial platform ladders, (five for Devon & Somerset and one for Cornwall) were simultaneously commissioned. The Taunton appliance is pictured prior to the line-up of all six appliances.

Rear cover: 25 April 2017 sees the Great Western Air Ambulance Charity's Helimed 65, registration G-GWAA, lift from outside Yate fire and ambulance stations, South Gloucestershire.

First published 2019

Amberley Publishing
The Hill, Stroud,
Gloucestershire, GL5 4EP

www.amberley-books.com

ISBN: 978 1 4456 8643 1 (print)
ISBN: 978 1 4456 8644 8 (ebook)

British Library Cataloguing in Publication Data.
A catalogue record for this book is available from the British Library.

Typeset in 10pt on 13pt Celeste.
Typesetting by Aura Technology and Software Services, India.
Printed in the UK.

Contents

The Author

Holding the Police Long Service and Good Conduct medal and retiring from the service in 1996, the author rose to the rank of chief superintendent in the Ministry of Defence Police after ten years' previous service in Avon & Somerset Constabulary. Married for fifty-two years with two daughters and seven grandchildren, he lives with his wife Margaret in Yate, South Gloucestershire. In 1999 he fulfilled a childhood ambition by learning to drive a bus, soon followed by several years as FIRST Group's regional accident investigator. To minimise blameworthy accidents he designed, and for many years presented, a successful accident prevention programme for the bus and coach industry in the Greater Bristol area. As a result he was honoured with the MBE in 2007. With a keen interest in photography and lifelong passion for all the emergency services, at seventy-one years of age he wrote his first book, *London's Emergency Service Vehicles,* a fully illustrated edition covering London's modern-day emergency services.

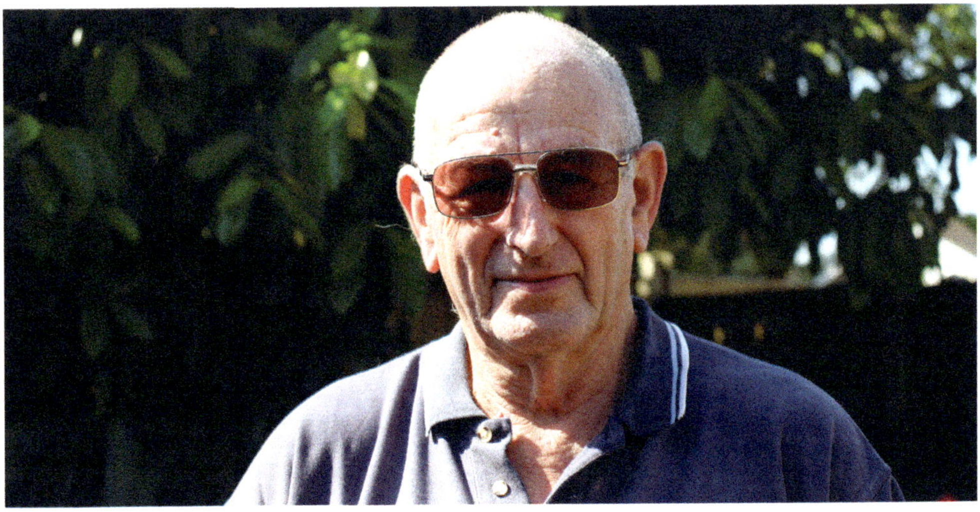

The author. (Image: Margaret Boulter)

Introduction

This book will appeal to all age groups and is written in non-technical terms. Nothing unpleasant is recorded, unmarked police vehicles do not knowingly appear, and the privacy of emergency service personnel and victims of accidents or crimes is not breached.

Vehicles are translated into the widest meaning of the word and cover land, sea and air in this vast geographical region stretching from South Gloucestershire to Cornwall, and from Weston-super-Mare to the Hampshire border.

Adopting a low profile to avoid distracting emergency service personnel and never using flash in any photographs, the author's preferred style of photography is action shots, often showing vehicles – blue light on – travelling at fairly high speeds in urban environments.

As the largest centre of population, the Bristol area naturally features prominently. However, every effort has been made to provide variety from across the region. All photographs are by the author unless otherwise stated. In the interest of historical accuracy all the images appearing in this book are 'as taken' with no attempt made to digitally alter, add or remove any aspect.

Aged seventy-three and wishing to record the knowledge I have for future generations, much of my information has been acquired over many years by personal contact, random jottings, social media and my own photography rather than consulting specific publications.

CHAPTER 1

Ambulance

Air Ambulances

Air ambulances, almost entirely funded by charitable donation, are based at six locations within the region. Those bases are at Newquay (Cornwall); Exeter and Eaglescott (both Devon); Henstridge (Dorset & Somerset); Almondsbury (Great Western); and Semington (Wiltshire). All fall within the massive geographical area, which also includes Gloucestershire and the Isles of Scilly, covered by the South Western Ambulance Service NHS Foundation Trust (SWASFT).

Backing up the crews of land-based emergency ambulances, air ambulances with their doctor, advanced paramedic trained personnel and specialised life-saving equipment, including blood, respond to potentially the most serious of incidents. For a variety of reasons, not least severe weather conditions, the air ambulance crew will sometimes attend in their dedicated critical care road vehicles, where necessary accompanying the land-based ambulance carrying the patient to the receiving hospital. Hospitals at Southmead (Bristol) and Derriford (Plymouth) are the region's designated adult major trauma centres (MTC), with Southampton General (Hampshire) being located just outside the eastern edge of the region. The Bristol Royal Hospital for Children (located adjacent to the Bristol Royal Infirmary) is the only children's MTC in the region.

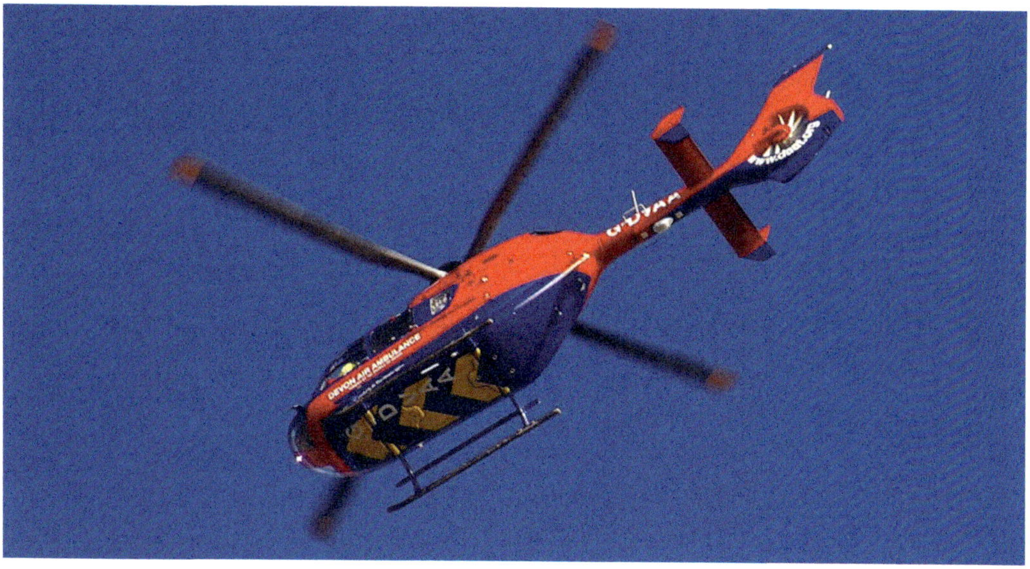

Devon air ambulance, registration G-DVAA, seen above Torquay. This aircraft is being replaced in mid-2020 by an Airbus H145, registration G-DAAS, which will be based in Exeter. The remaining Devon air ambulance, G-DAAN, will then transfer to their other base at Eaglescott near Great Torrington. 2009.

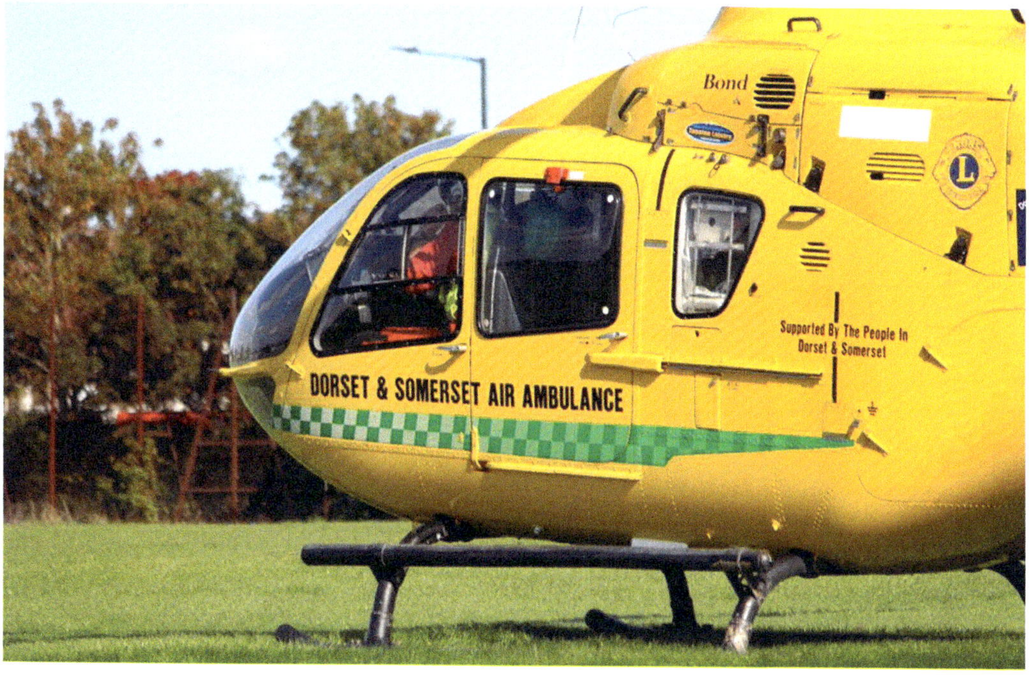

With the helipad at the Southmead Hospital MTC already occupied, the designated overspill site at the nearby Horfield Leisure Centre was used. On an exceptionally busy day, the departure of the Dorset & Somerset helicopter was immediately followed by the arrival at the Leisure Centre of a Devon aircraft. 26 September 2015.

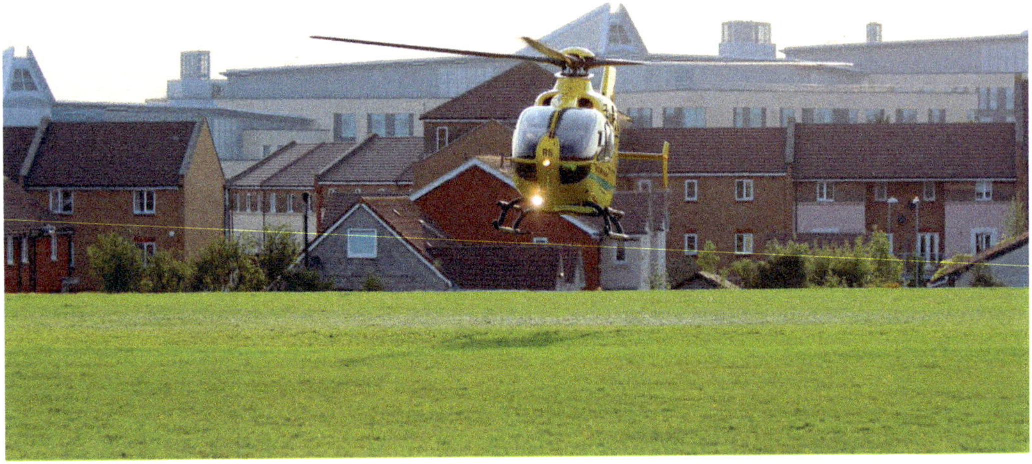

On this occasion the Dorset & Somerset air ambulance, G-DORS, call sign Helimed 10, again features at Horfield Leisure Centre. Southmead Hospital is visible in the background. The hospital helipad was clear at that moment, but by prior arrangement it remained that way for the Great Western air ambulance arriving a few minutes later to fly direct to the hospital with a more critical patient. 12 May 2016.

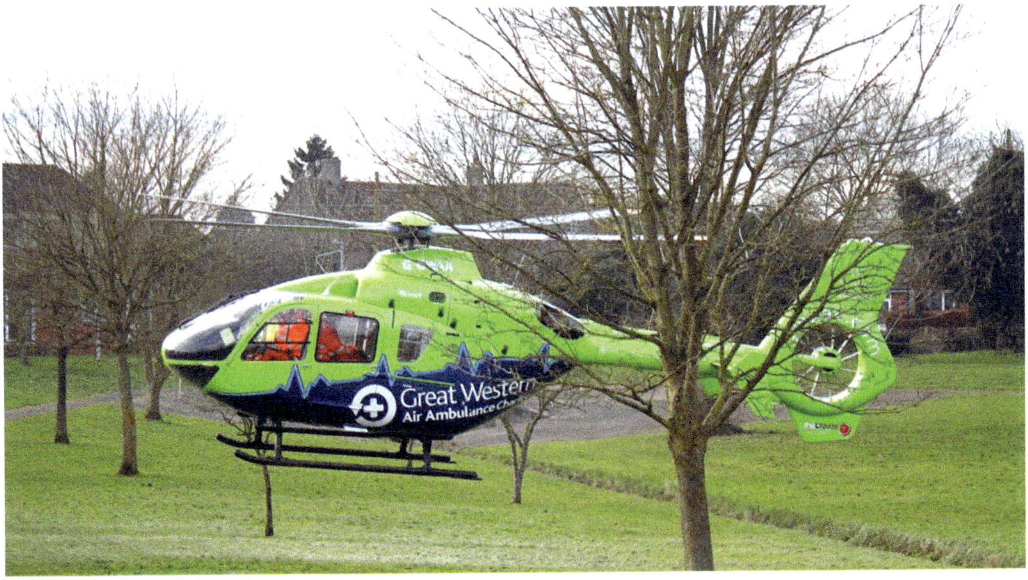

While requiring a great deal of skill by the pilot and observation by the crew in daylight, it is easy to appreciate that at night the obstacles created by trees could make landing in unfamiliar territory extremely hazardous and the use of night-vision equipment essential. In this emergency, G-GWAA is pictured lifting from Brimsham Park, Yate. The helicopter was replaced in 2017 by G-GWAC, a very similar model in identical livery but fitted with a longer range fuel tank. 20 January 2015. (Image: John Lockwood)

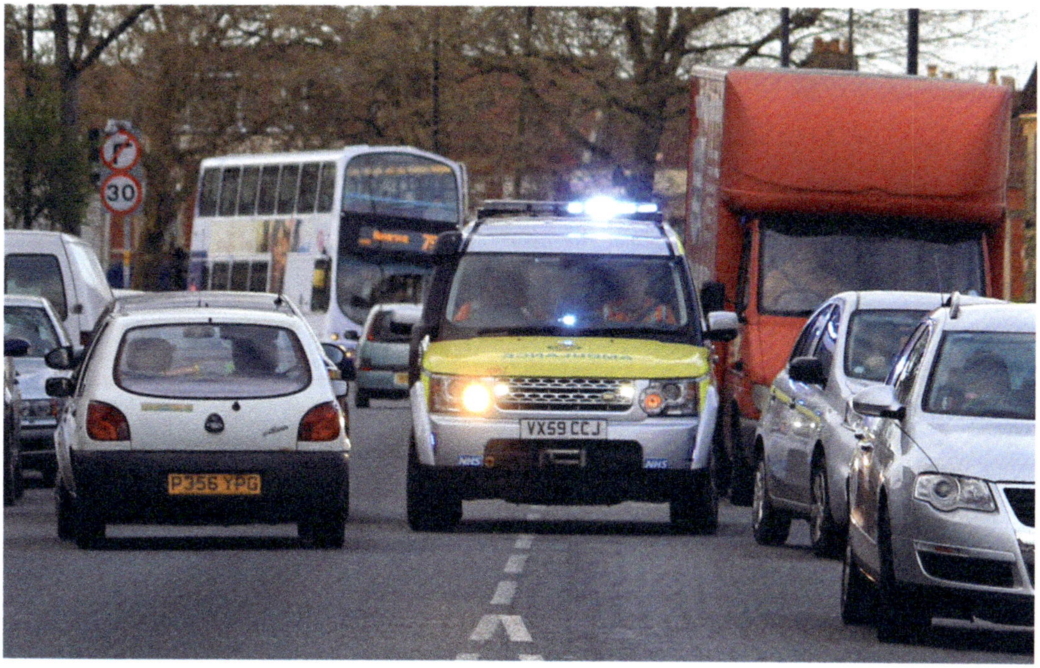

Accelerating hard, this long-range photograph from the sanctuary of a traffic island some 300 metres distant captures the Great Western Air Ambulance Charity (GWAAC) Land Rover Discovery VX59 CCJ responding down Gloucester Road as it heads towards central Bristol. 17 April 2015.

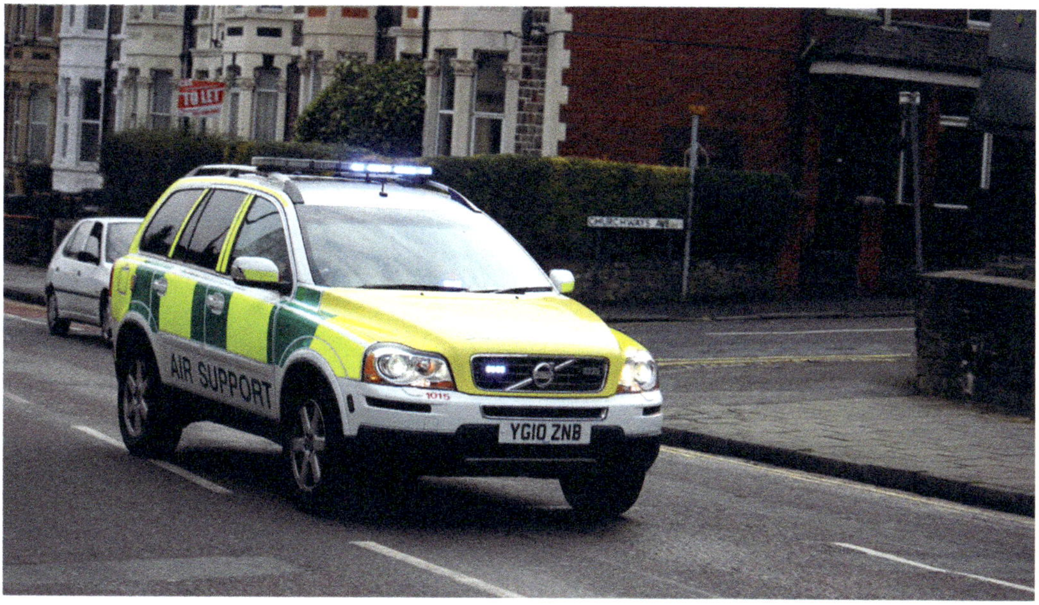

The other regular GWAAC land-based vehicle is Volvo YG10 ZNB, which is captured passing Churchways Avenue, Bristol 7, as it responds on the blues and twos in the Horfield Common direction. The wording on the side has subsequently been altered from 'Air Support' to read 'Critical Care'. 13 March 2015.

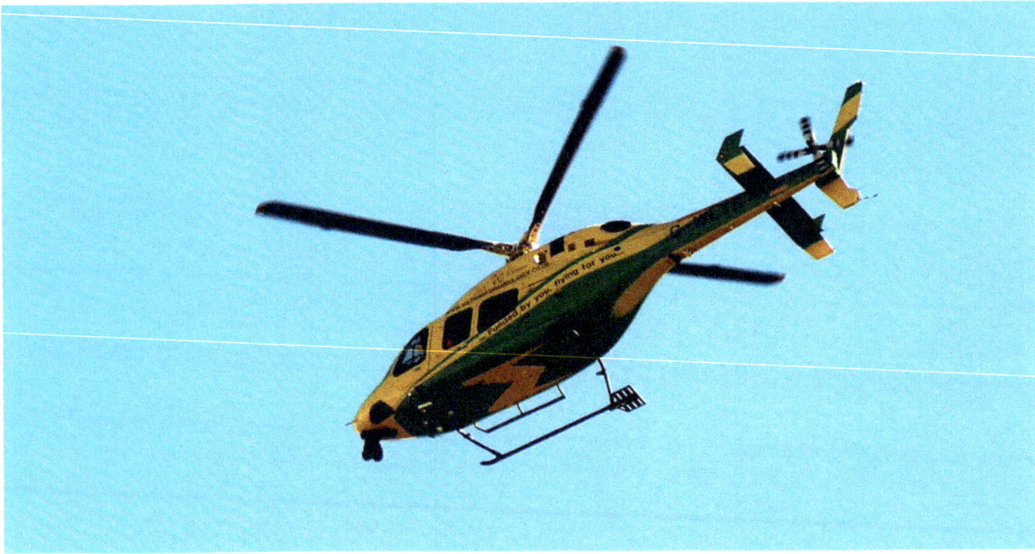

Wiltshire's air ambulance is Helimed 22, registration G-WLTS, a Bell 429 with a top speed of 178 mph and able to reach anywhere in the county within eleven minutes from its base at Semington near Melksham, which opened in late May 2018. July 2016.

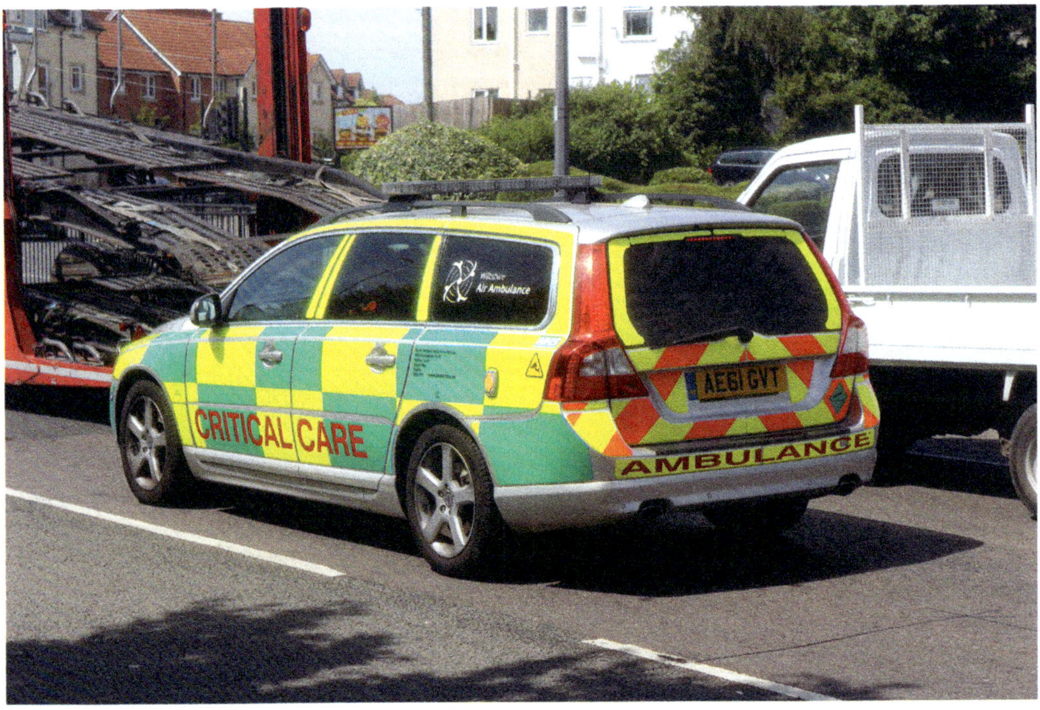

Wiltshire's land-based response vehicle on this date is Volvo estate AE61 GVT, seen at routine road speed in Filton, South Gloucestershire probably having just left the neighbouring GWAAC base. The Filton facility moved on 16 October 2018 to a new base adjacent to the M4/M5 interchange. 7 July 2017.

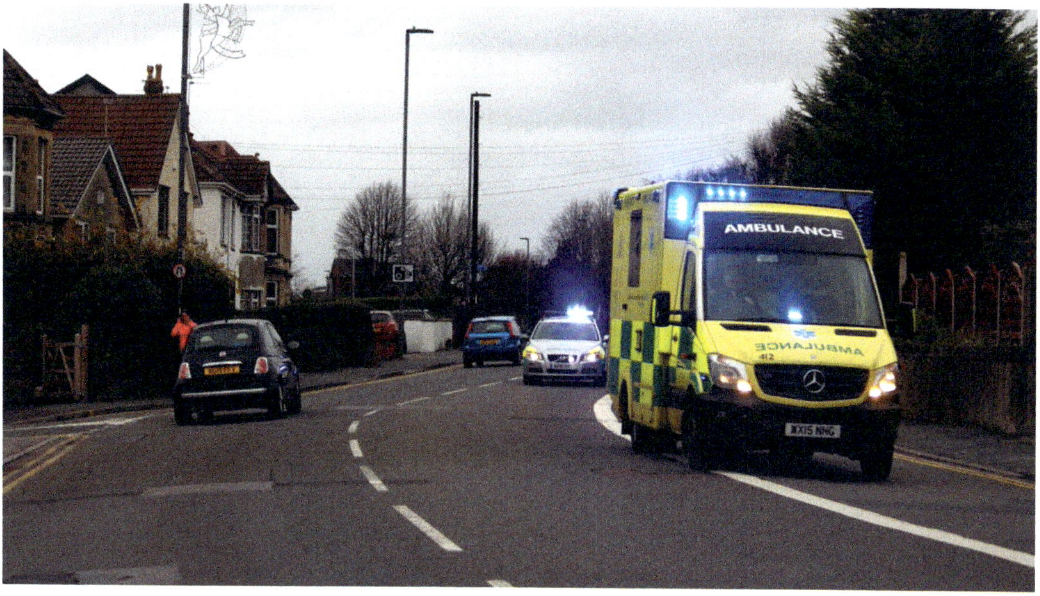

At high speed, both vehicles on the blues and twos, a Bath-based ambulance races along Gloucester Road North towards Southmead Hospital, Bristol, with the Critical Care Wiltshire Volvo estate close behind. 5 December 2015.

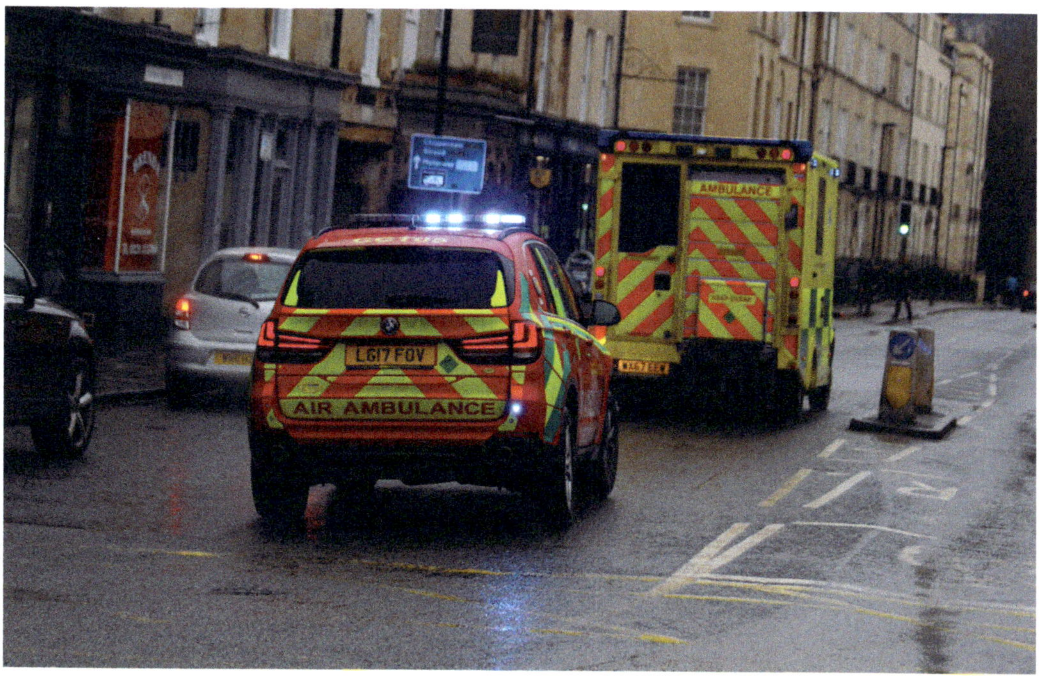

In absolutely dreadful weather conditions, with a very low cloud base and continuous swirling drizzle, a SWASFT ambulance is closely followed by air ambulance Critical Care BMW X5 demonstrator LG17 FOV, which was in the region during the latter part of 2017 and early 2018. It was captured on film entering Bathwick Street, Bath. 20 January 2018.

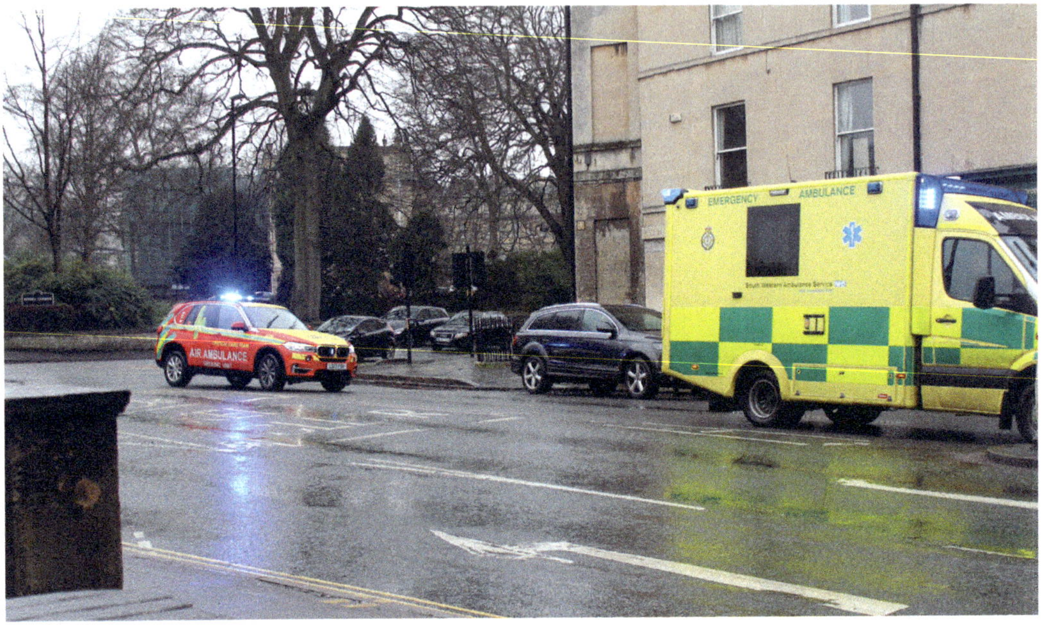

My grandson Jamie was across the junction and able to capture this view of the vehicles from Bathwick Street. 20 January 2018. (Image: Jamie Enright)

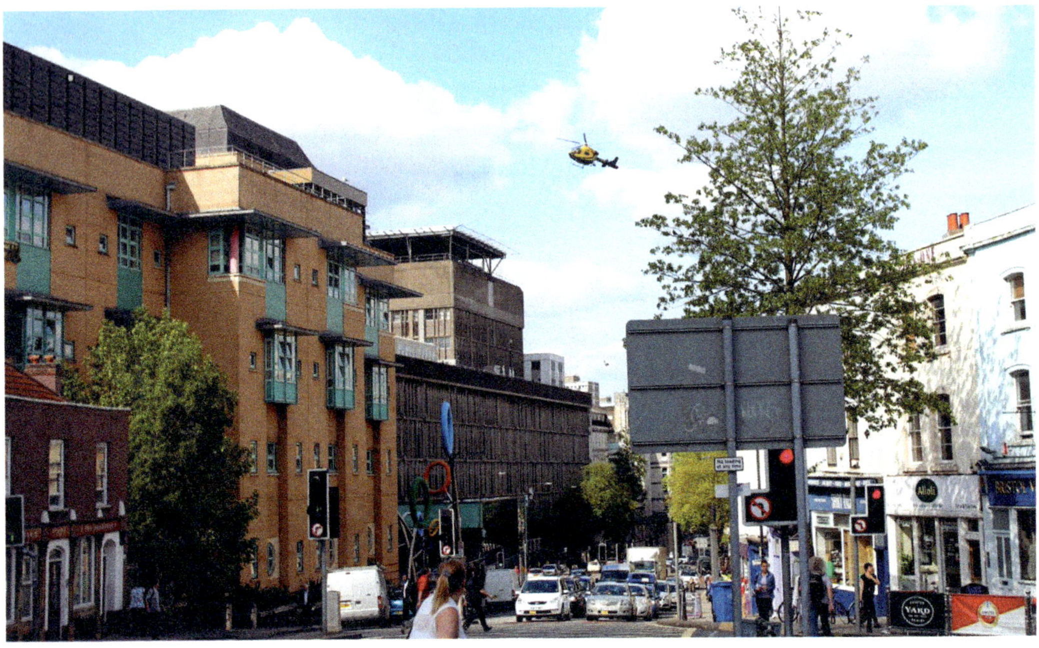

A general view down Upper Maudlin Street, Bristol. The rooftop Bristol Royal Infirmary helipad is about to be visited by the then Wiltshire joint Police/Ambulance helicopter, G-WPAS. This helicopter left service at the end of December 2014 when the new Wiltshire air ambulance, G-WLTS, commenced operating independently. The modern building to the left of the picture is Bristol Royal Hospital for Children, the Paediatric MTC for the entire West of England. 15 May 2014.

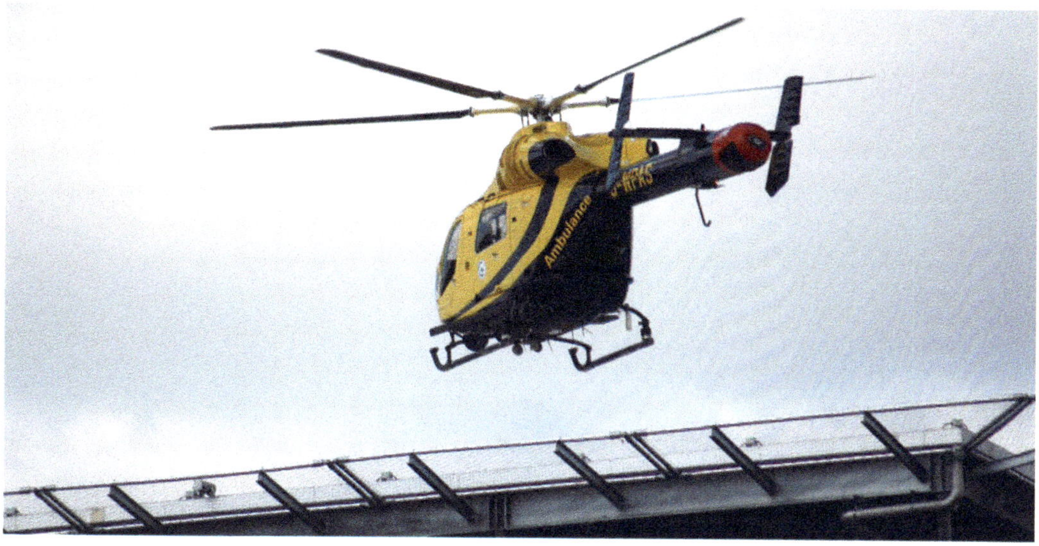

On lifting from the helipad, helicopters generally fly backwards. Should there be a malfunction the pilot can clearly see the safe landing spot he or she has just lifted from, thus making for a safer return to the helipad. This is particularly important if it is a rooftop structure, such as the one at the Bristol Royal Infirmary, located some 200 feet above ground. Rooftop structures also benefit from the presence of on-site firefighters on the helipad, who can deploy instantly in the event of a flight emergency many floors above street level. 15 May 2014.

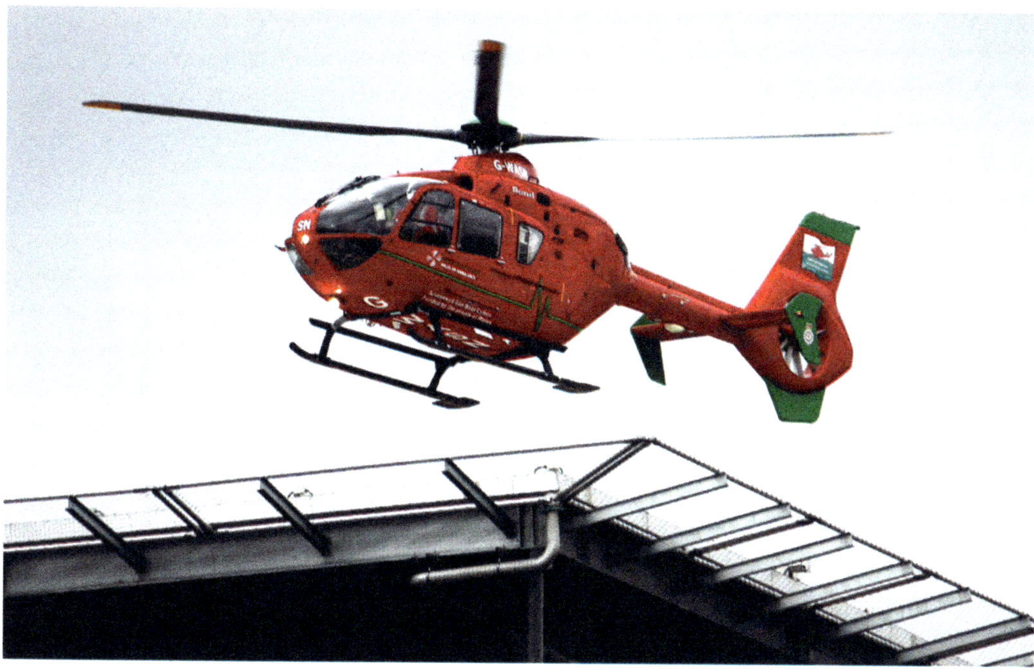

Cardiff-based Welsh air ambulance G-WASN, call sign Helimed 67, is pictured lifting off from the roof of the Bristol Royal Infirmary helipad. At the time there was no adult or paediatric MTC in Wales. 28 February 2015.

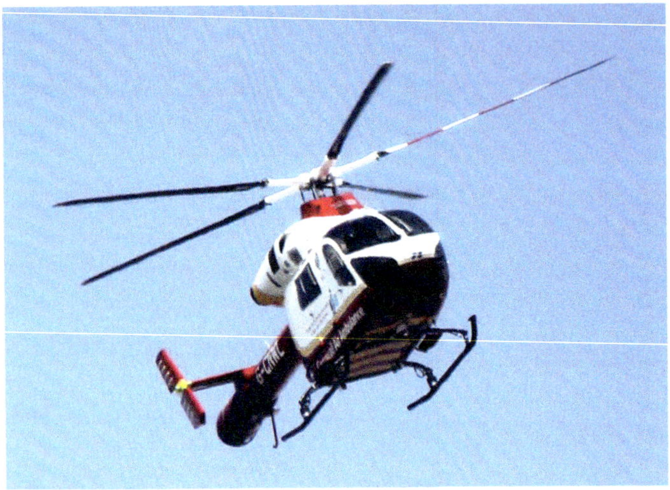

Last, but by no means least, in this selection of air ambulance images is Cornwall's G-CNWL, based at Newquay, which is seen on approach to Southmead Hospital. This may well be a first landing at this venue for this aircraft as Derriford Hospital, the Plymouth MTC, is geographically much nearer to the Cornish aircraft's main operating area. Early April 2015.

Alcohol Recovery Centre

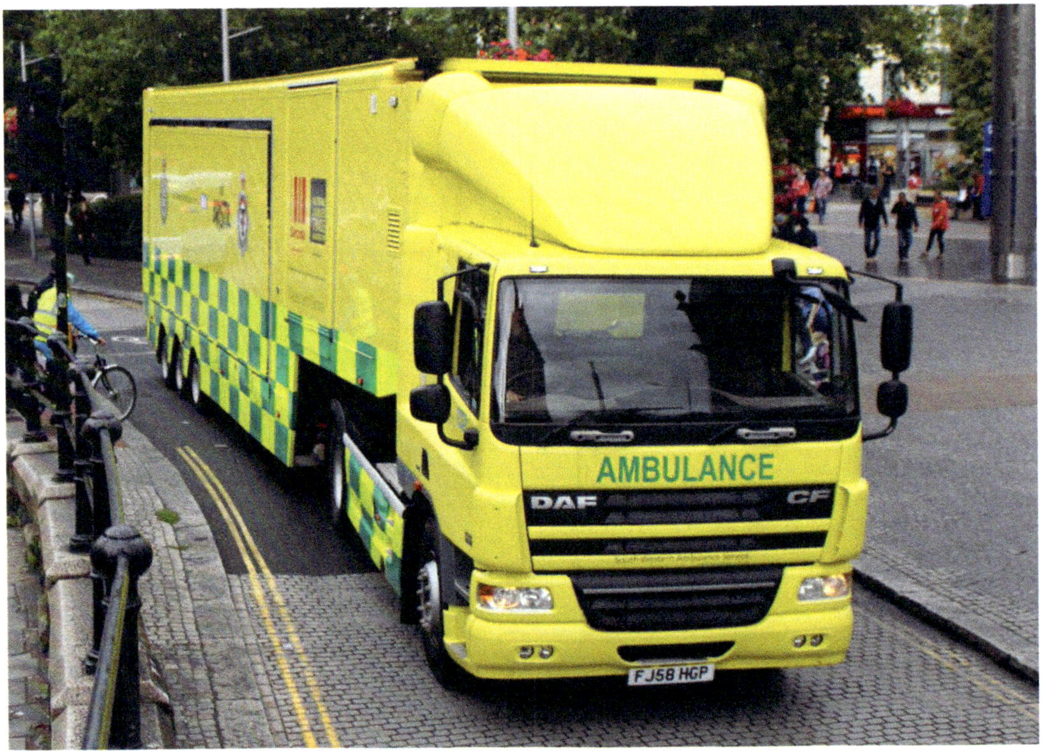

More commonly known as the ARC, the unit in its original guise is pictured crossing Bristol city centre prior to setting up for weekend evenings adjacent to City Hall. The existence of this vehicle helps in reducing numbers of late-night revellers needing to go to Accident & Emergency for minor treatment. Following an engine blow out to FJ58 HGP, Royal Mail now provide motive power from their fleet of articulated prime movers and their logo now appears on the sides of the trailer, as does the wording 'Mobile Treatment Centre'. 14 August 2015.

Avon & Somerset Search & Rescue

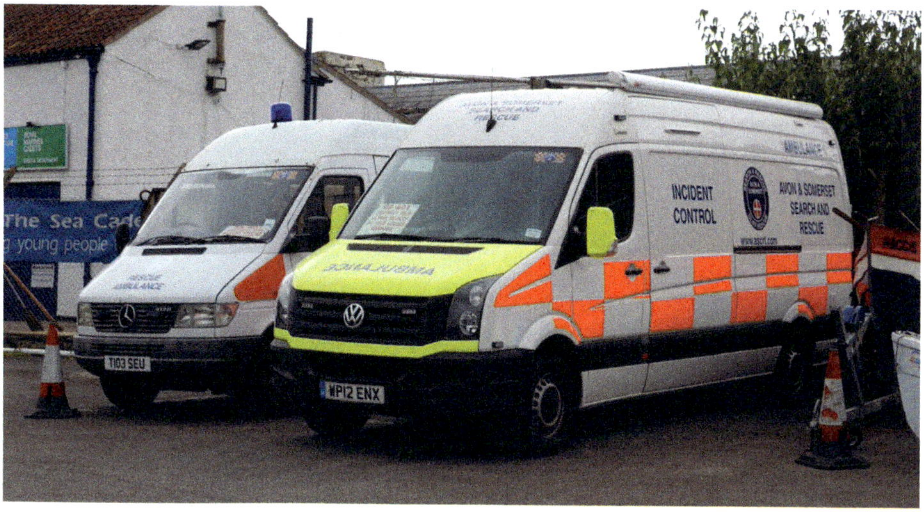

A well-established voluntary organisation, Avon & Somerset Search & Rescue members provide valuable assistance to the emergency services. Some members are experienced rope specialists, a particularly useful feature with the Avon Gorge on their doorstep and Cheddar Gorge around 20 miles away in adjoining Somerset. Mobilised via Avon & Somerset Constabulary, the vehicles are marked as ambulances, hence their inclusion in this section of the book. 4 July 2016.

British Red Cross

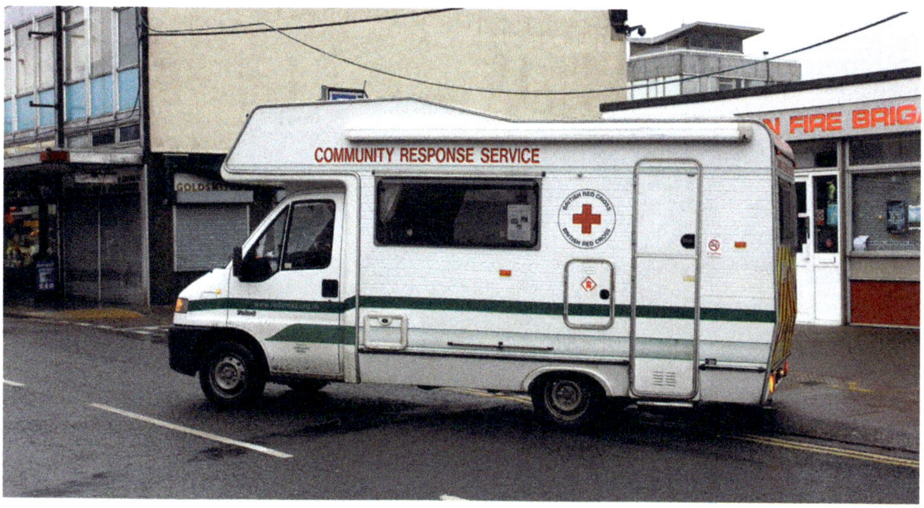

No blue lights or siren on this British Red Cross vehicle mobilising from its base at Keynsham fire station in north-east Somerset. This service is also manned by volunteers, to whom tribute is paid, as it is to numerous voluntary organisations throughout the region. The title Community Response Service has undergone several name changes and is now known as the Fire & Emergency Support Service. 13 November 1997.

Command, Control and Communications

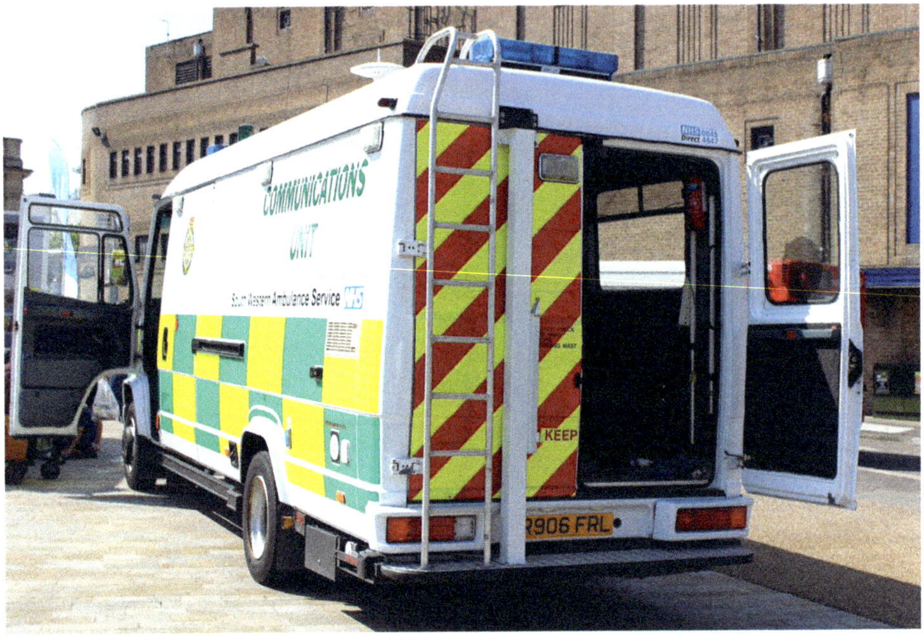

A superb display of 999 vehicles was present on Taunton's Castle Green in an event open to the public hosted by Avon & Somerset Constabulary. A SWASFT Communications Unit was in attendance, map boards inside featuring the vehicle's forthcoming deployment to Dorset's four-day Bournemouth Air Festival being held later that week. 17 August 2015.

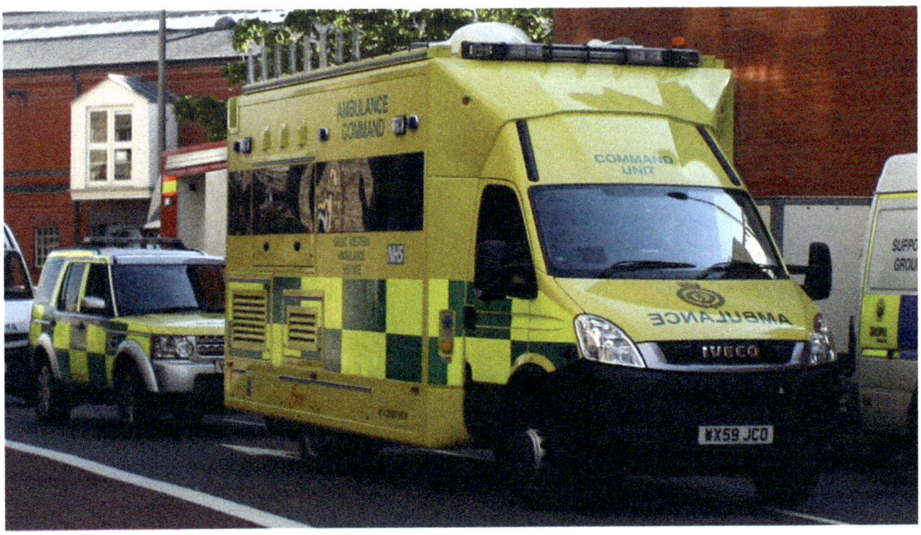

Anchor Road, Bristol. The SWASFT Iveco Command Unit, WX59 JCO, awaits instructions to move forward at a major chemical incident exercise. In a much appreciated gesture, the general public were welcome to observe the exercise attended by over forty front-line emergency vehicles. This unit has subsequently become a Clinical Simulation Vehicle. 2 October 2011.

Emergency Ambulances

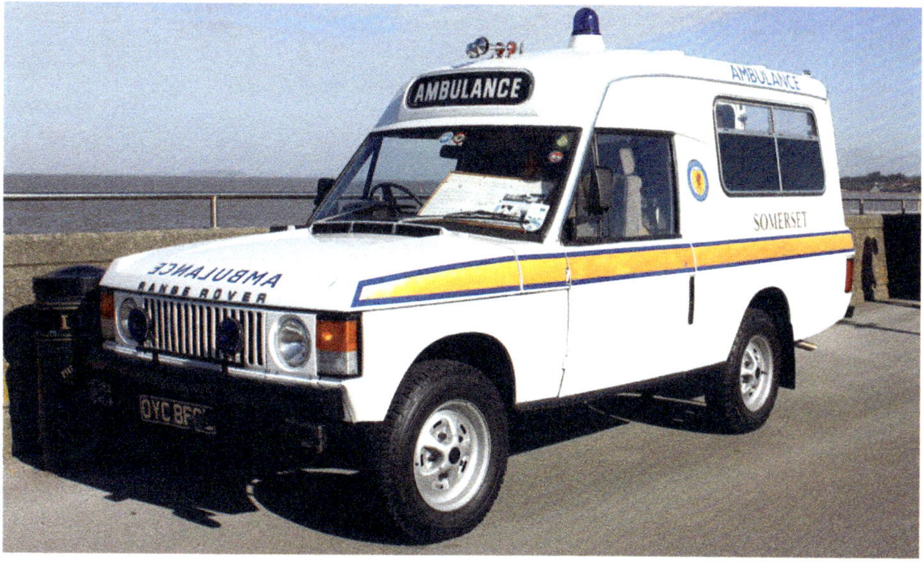

A real gem from the past that appeared at the Burnham-on-Sea Rescue Day was this 1973 Somerset Ambulance Service Range Rover, OYC 860L, which was preserved in first-class condition despite its age. 31 August 2014.

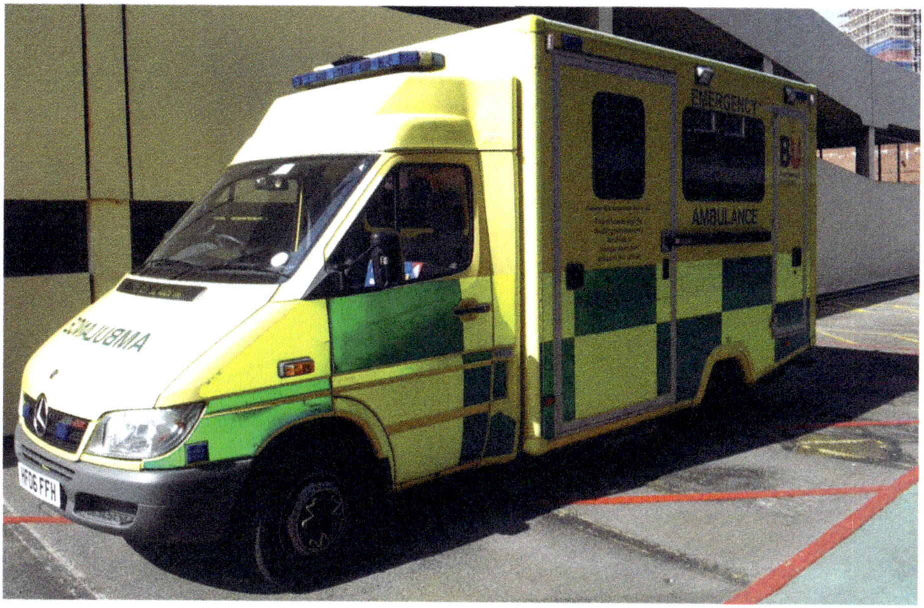

Courtesy of a 2014 donation from the South Western Ambulance Service NHS Foundation Trust (SWASFT), Bournemouth University uses this static Mercedes Sprinter/WAS ambulance, registration HF06 FFH, as a skills laboratory for working in a restricted environment in realistic situations. This is as part of their BSc (Hons) three-year full-time course in Paramedic Science. (Image: Paul Billett)

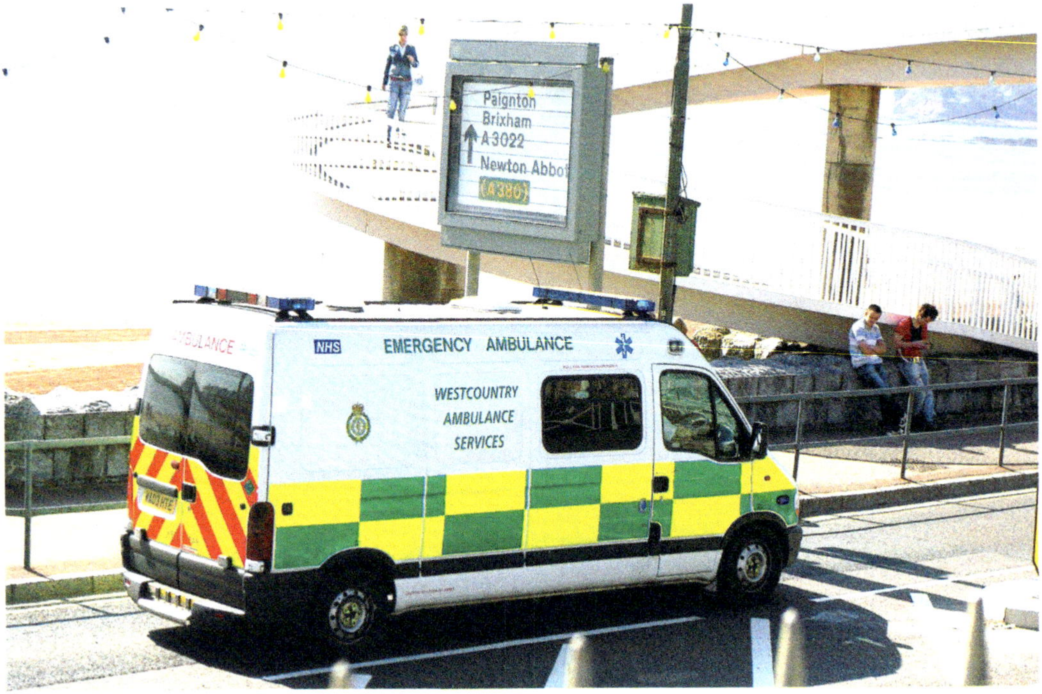

Bearing the former West Country Ambulance Services logo, this Renault ambulance, WA03 HTE, makes its way to an emergency along a very sunny Torquay seafront. 2011.

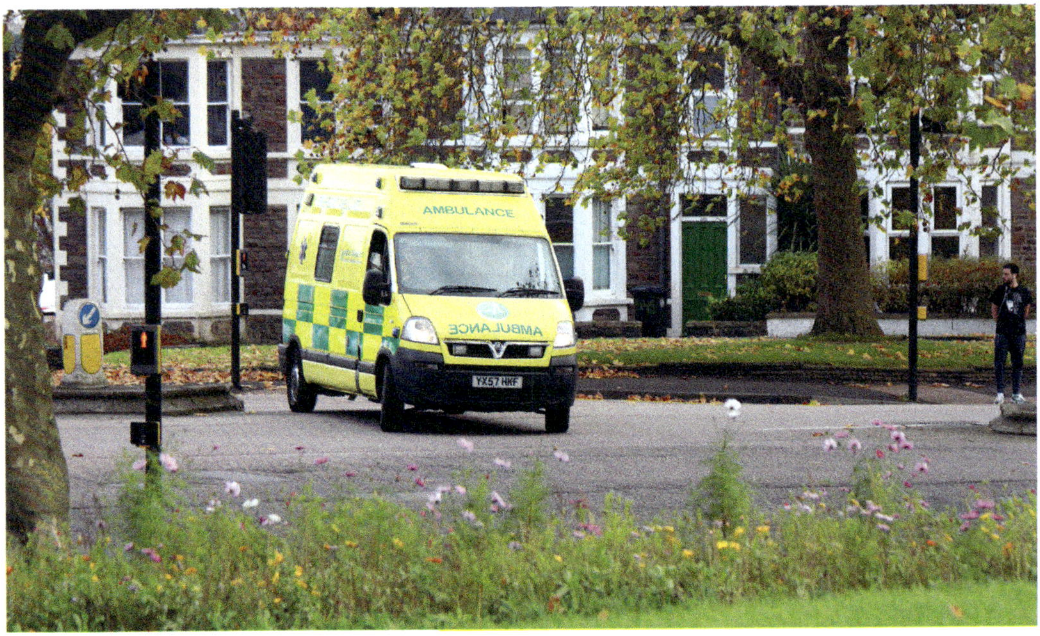

Bristol Ambulance Emergency Medical Service YX57 HKF turns at the top of Muller Road in a picturesque autumnal setting as it makes its way towards nearby Southmead Hospital. 28 October 2017.

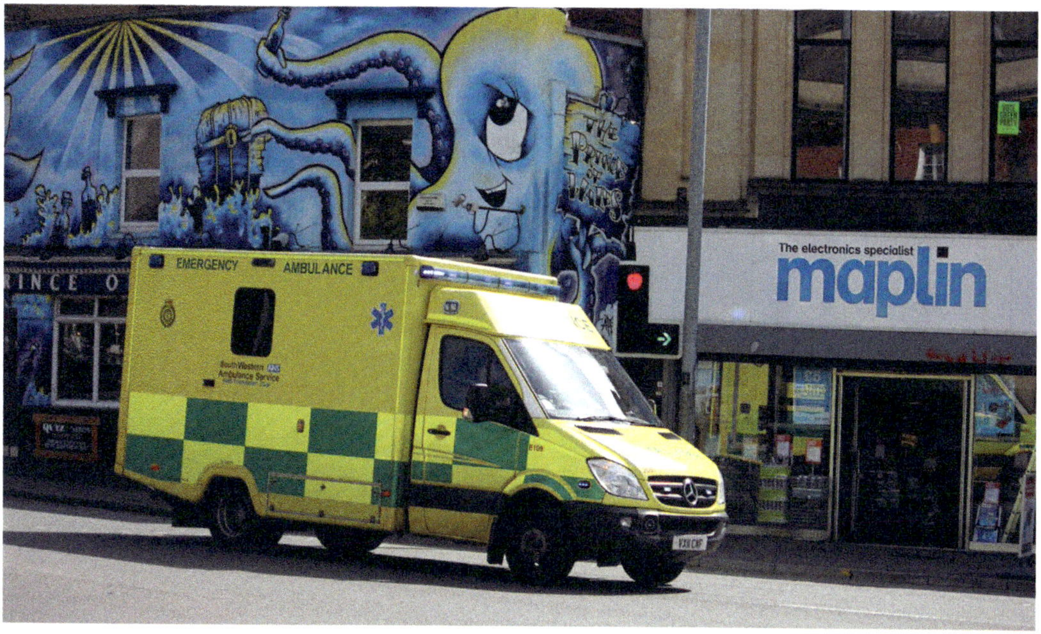

Contrasts in blue as SWASFT ambulance VX11 CNF, seen on an emergency response with the older style forward-facing light bar above the cab, passes the distinctive façade to the Prince of Wales public house and the former Maplin store at the Zetland Road junction, Bristol. 16 May 2015.

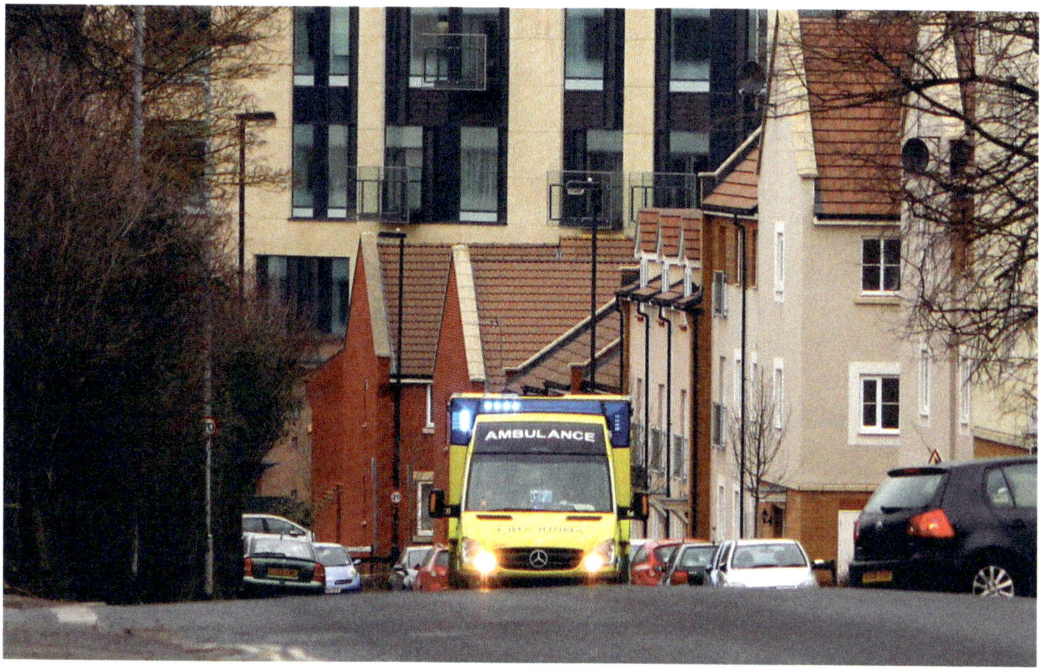

Displaying the larger array of blue lights surrounding the top of the vehicle cab, WN63 BYC climbs Dorian Road on a shout, the distinctive lines of Southmead Hospital dominating the background. 6 February 2015.

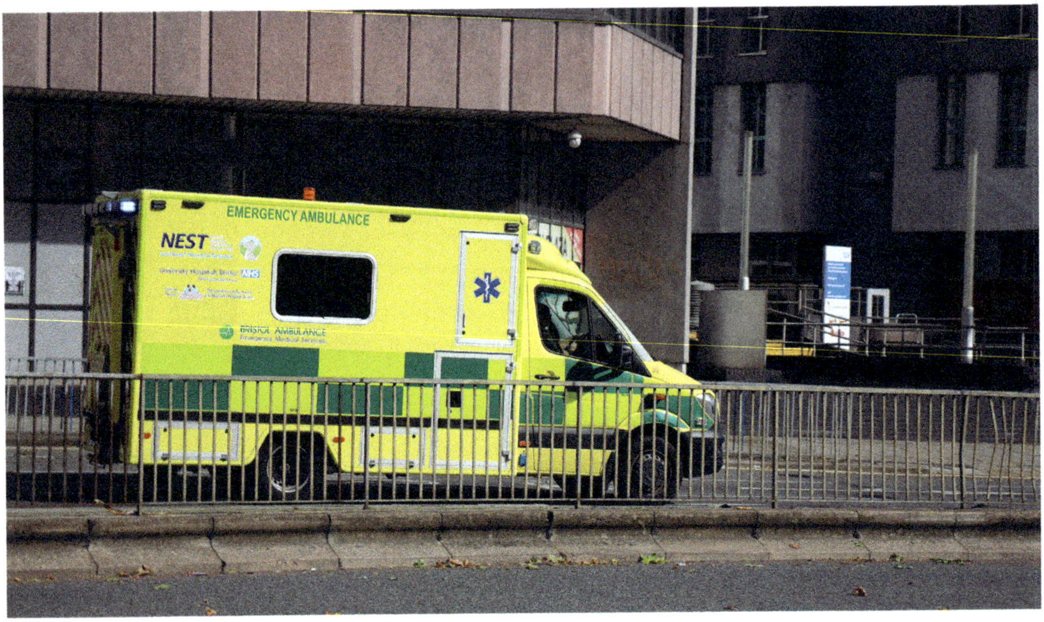

Based at St Michael's Hospital, Bristol, a Newborn Emergency Stabilisation & Transport Team (NEST) ambulance, CN18 AZO, operated by Bristol Ambulance Emergency Medical Services on behalf of the NHS, heads outbound on the blue light from central Bristol. This may well be a lengthy journey in the upper part of the region, with specialists onboard to assist the baby, involving transfer to the most appropriate neonatal hospital. A second transport team run by Peninsular Neonatal Transport Service are based at Derriford Hospital, Plymouth, primarily to respond in the lower part of the of the region covered by this book. 19 September 2018.

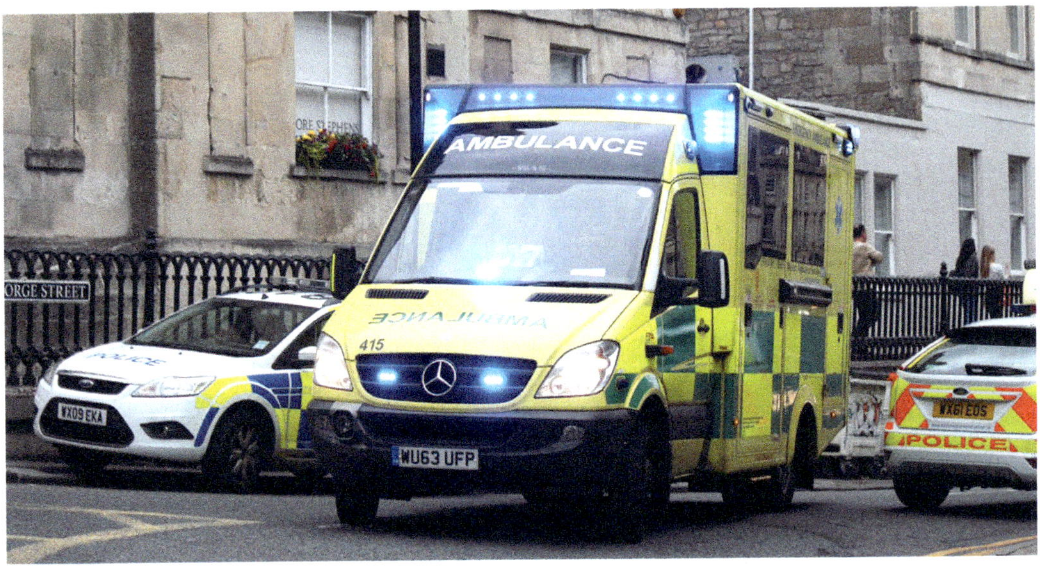

With a vivid array of forward-facing blue lights, locally based ambulance WU63 UFP squeezes between two police units dealing with a separate public disorder incident in George Street, Bath. 27 June 2015.

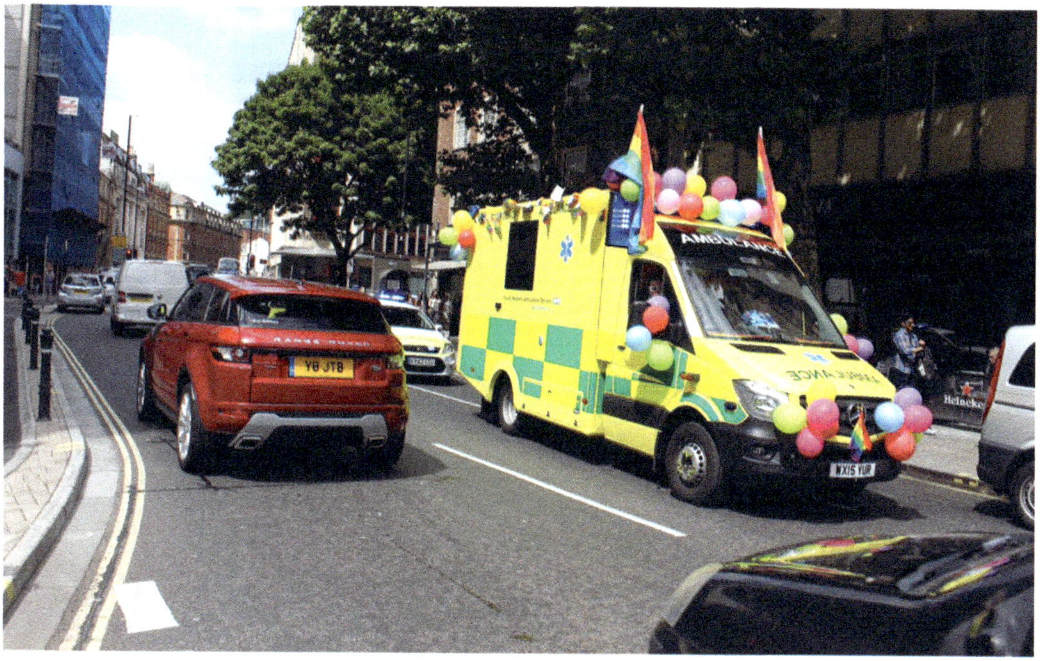

Equality, inclusiveness and diversity to the fore, SWASFT ambulance WX15 YUR makes its way up Baldwin Street, Bristol, towards Castle Green as part of the annual Pride festival. 11 July 2015.

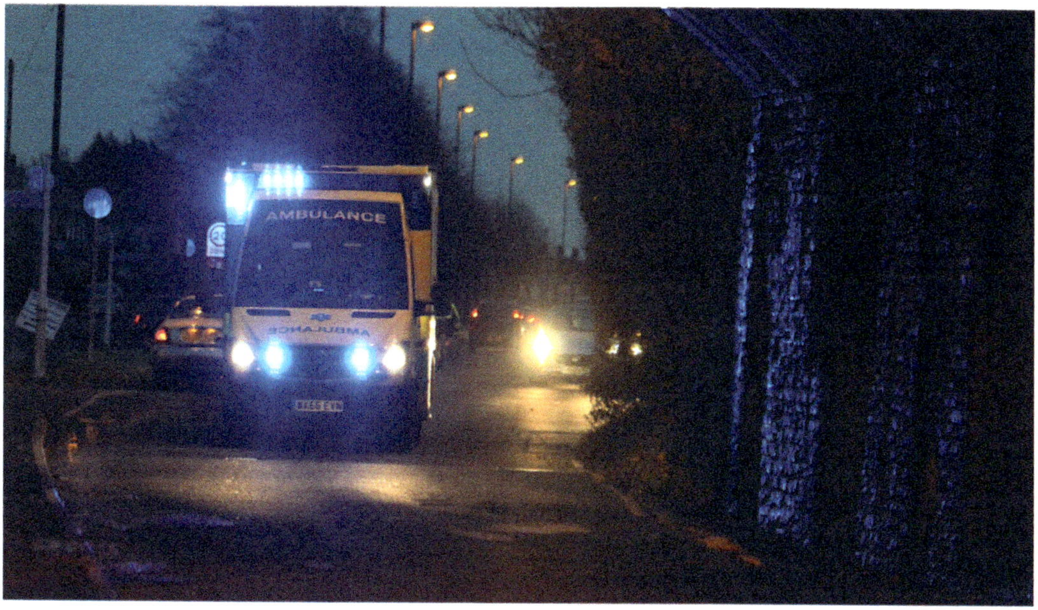

On hearing a distant siren but not knowing where it was coming from at that stage, given the restricted width of the roadway in Gypsy Patch Lane, the author brought his vehicle to a halt. Within seconds blue reflections were seen in the distance, culminating in the fast approach of WX66 EVN and the capture of this distinctive image by the author's wife. 22 November 2017. (Image: Margaret Boulter)

Hazardous Area Response Team (HART)

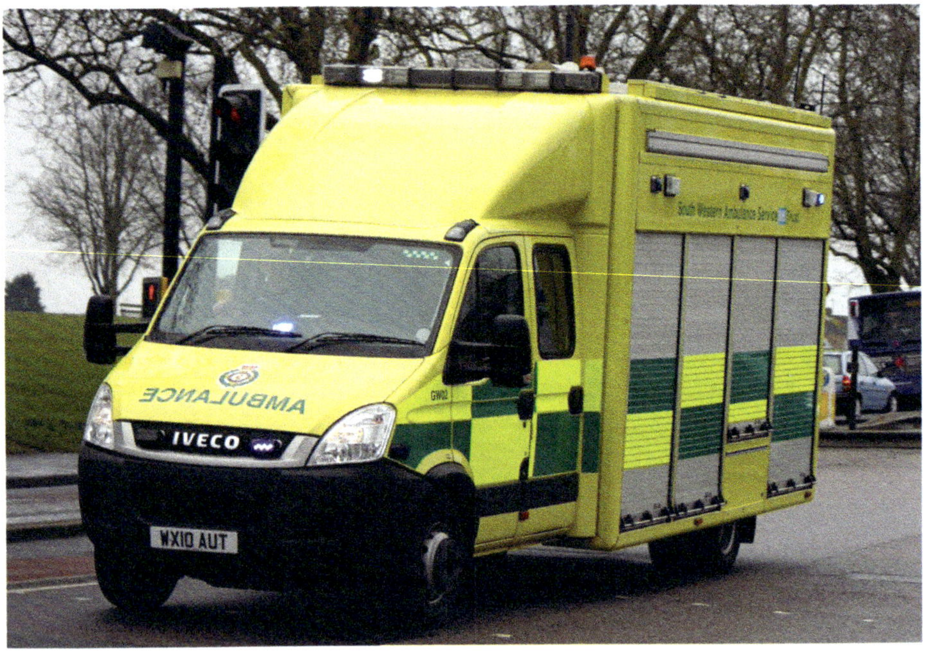

Established in 2010, HART teams in the region covered by this book are based on the outskirts of Bristol and in Exeter. HART are specially trained paramedics who have additional skills enabling them, as the name suggests, to go into the most hazardous of situations such as building collapses, fast-flowing water, noxious substances, road traffic collision entrapments, or working at height to stabilise the patient while other agencies such as the fire and rescue service use their specialist equipment and knowledge to actually free the patient. 13 March 2015.

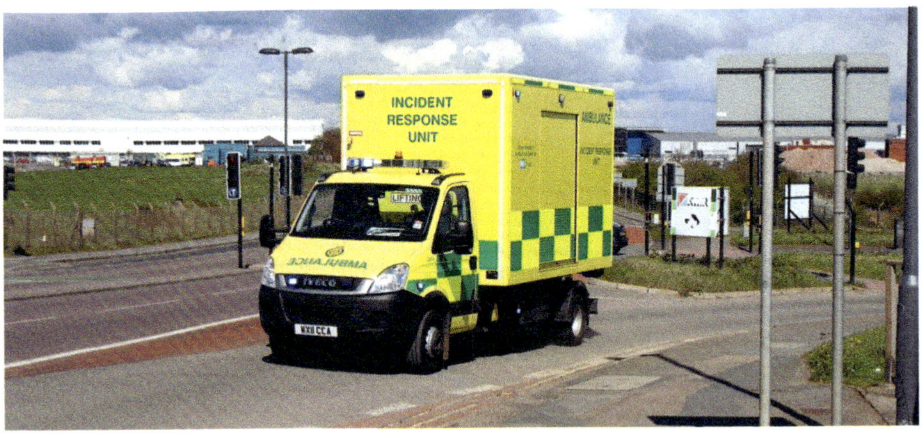

Used to transport the Bristol-based Polaris six-wheel drive vehicle, which enables difficult terrain to be crossed, Iveco WX11 CCA has just left its Filton base in South Gloucestershire and heads towards Bristol. In this first generation design the box section is hydraulically unloaded to ground level and the Polaris driven out. 11 April 2012.

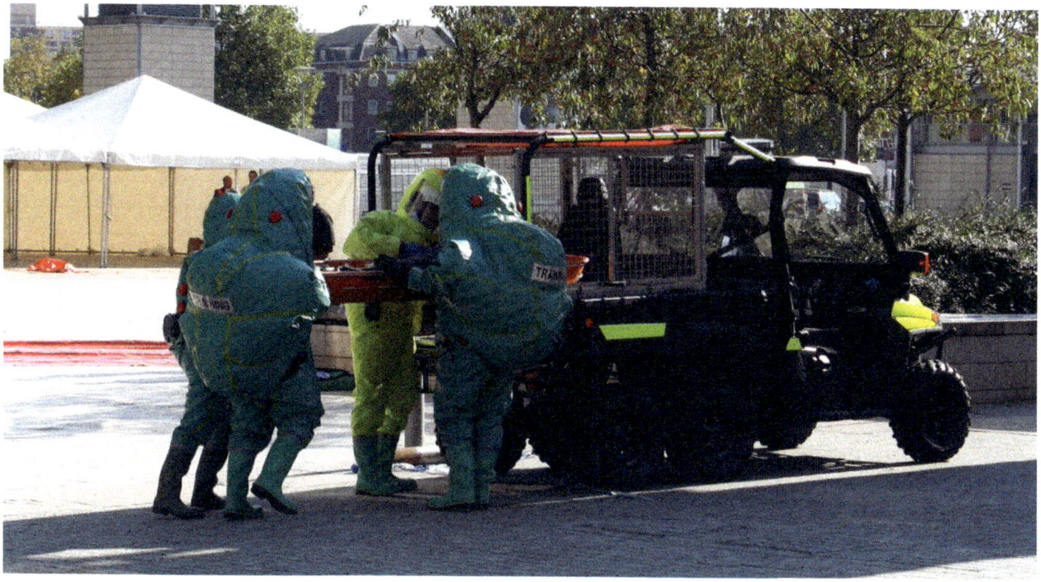

The HART Polaris in action at a major incident chemical exercise in Millennium Square, Bristol. The cumbersome gas-tight suits are marked 'Training' but use of their operational suits was only too real in Salisbury following the poisoning on 4 March 2018 of two Russian citizens and a police officer attending the scene. While they all survived, in the subsequent incident in nearby Amesbury on 30 June 2018 two people succumbed to innocently handling a discarded container, as a result of which Dawn Sturgess, forty-four years old, sadly died eight days later. 2 October 2011.

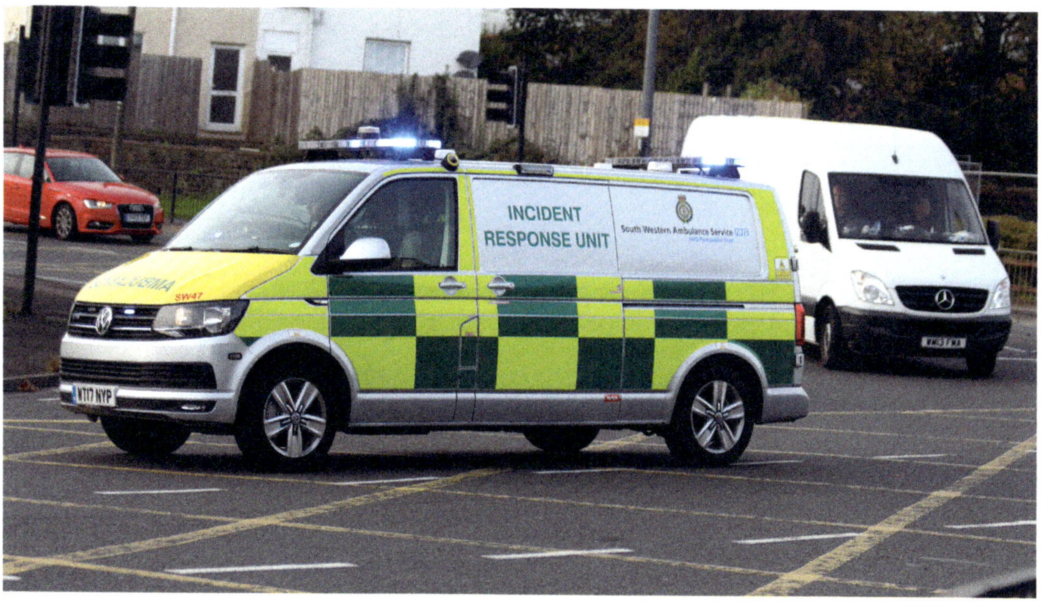

The latest wave of HART Incident Response Unit vehicles introduced in the Bristol area in late 2017 include three VWs identical in outward appearance. One of them, WT17 NYP, is pictured negotiating Filton roundabout. 1 November 2017.

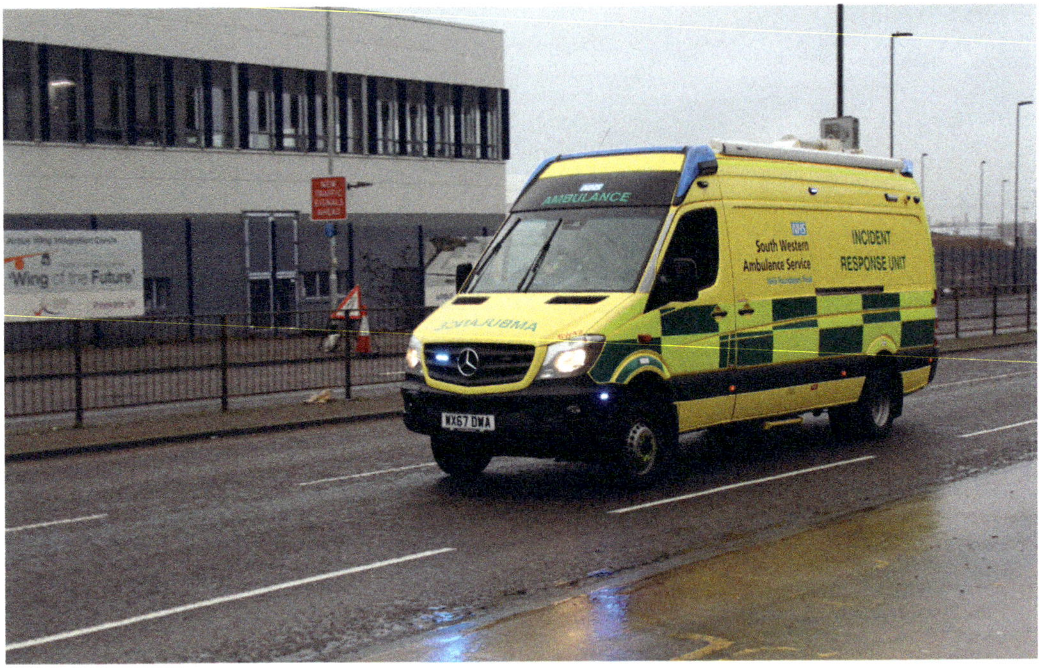

In constant drizzle, WX67 DWA, one of three larger Mercedes Sprinter HART vehicles now based at North Bristol Park, South Gloucestershire, is pictured soon after having mobilised from its nearby base. 28 January 2018. (Image: Margaret Boulter)

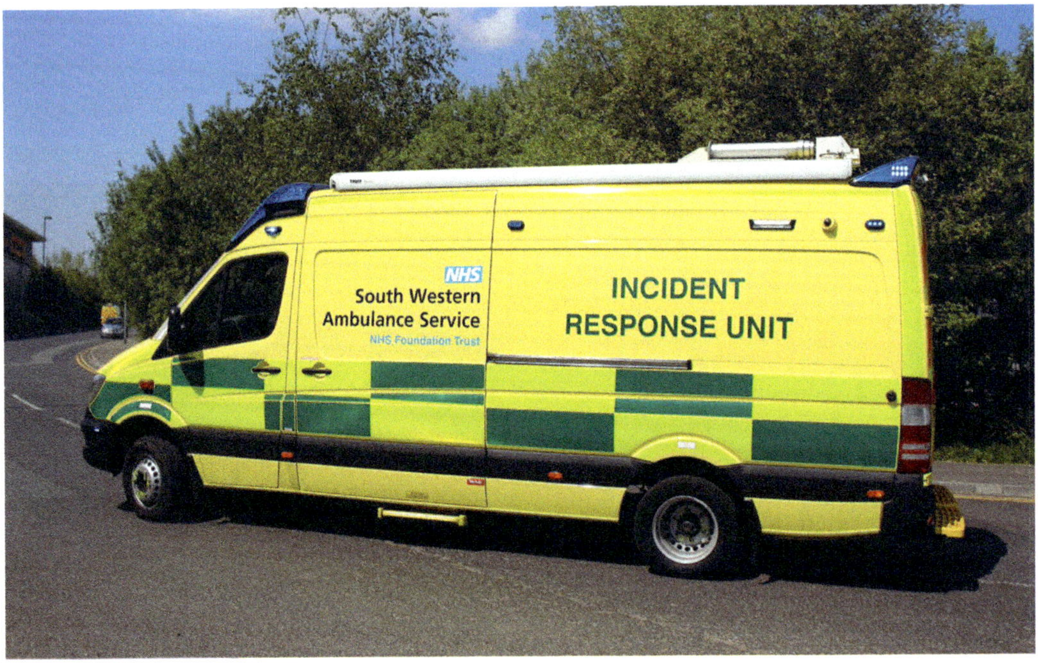

A two-vehicle HART turnout saw larger Incident Response Units WX67 DWA (in the distance) and WX67 DWC (nearest camera) go mobile on the blues from their Filton base. 19 May 2018.

Jumbulances

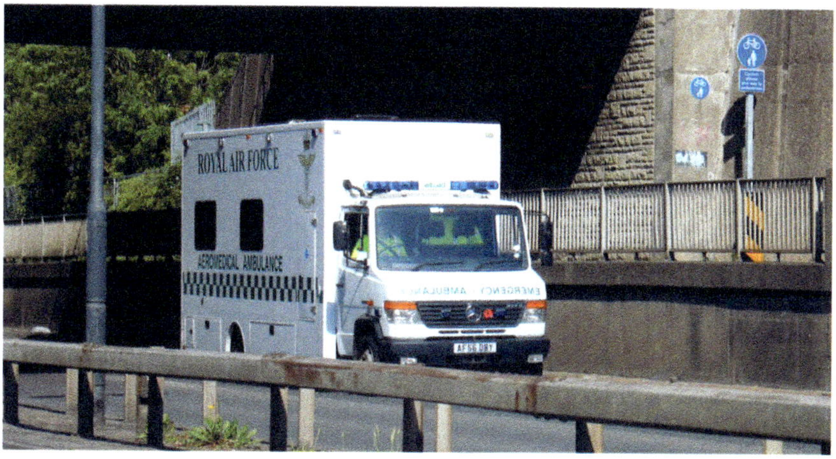

Known as a Jumbulance because of its size – albeit it remains marked as an ambulance – readers may recognise this unique RAF Aeromedical ambulance as the one seen on television under heavy police escort when it was used to transport the Scottish Ebola victim Pauline Cafferkey from a North London airfield to the Royal London Free Hospital in October 2015. However, on the weekend these images were shot its size was used to great advantage in transporting intensive care patients and their complex life-saving equiment across Bristol from the closing Frenchay Hospital to the brand-new Southmead Hospital. It is pictured on the A4174 Avon Ring Road at Abbey Wood when heading back to Frenchay for its next patient. 17 May 2014. (Image: Margaret Boulter)

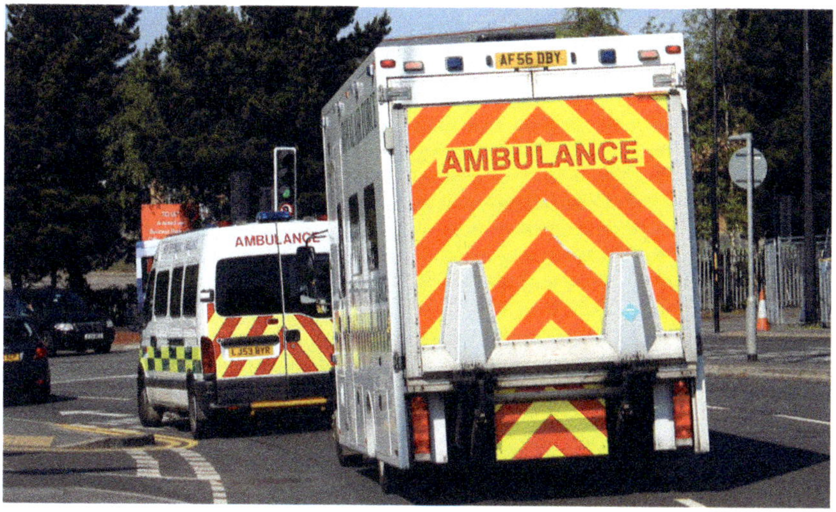

The considerable size of the Jumbulance is evident from this comparison shot of a conventional high-dependancy ambulance as both vehicles head down Southmead Road, South Gloucestershire, near to the Bristol boundary. Apparently very few Jumbulances of this size, or slightly smaller but marked as a Jumbulance, exist in the UK although the Jumbulance Trust do operate coaches designed to carry the disabled. 18 May 2014. (Image: Margaret Boulter)

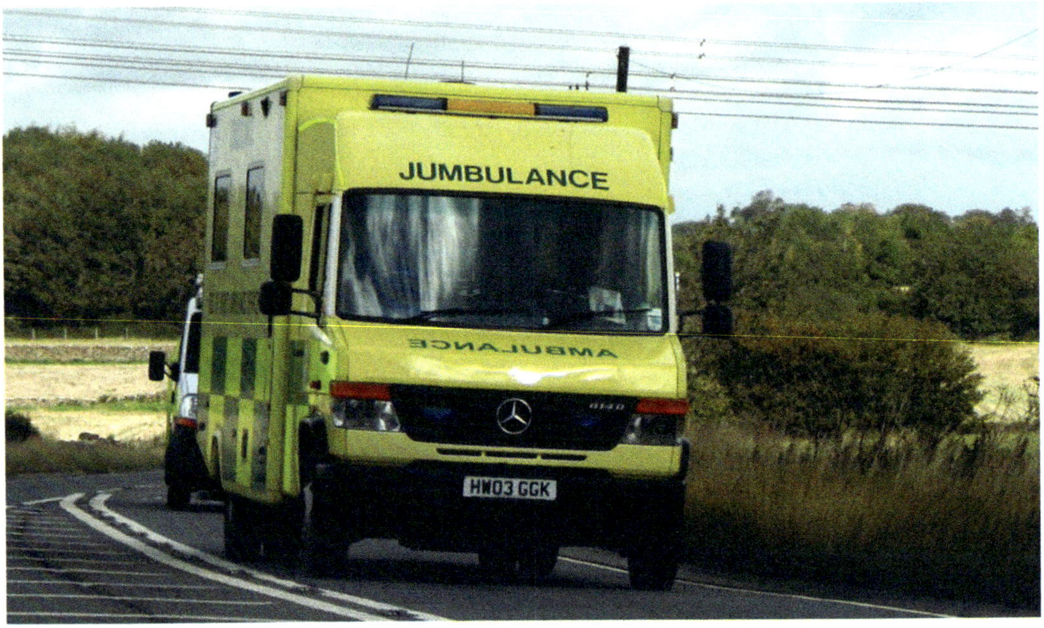

An extremely rare sight coming the opposite way on the A46 Tormarton–Bath road near Junction 18 of the M4 was Mercedes 814D, registration HW03 GGK, a Jumbulance also marked ambulance belonging to the Isle of Wight Ambulance Service. September 2012.

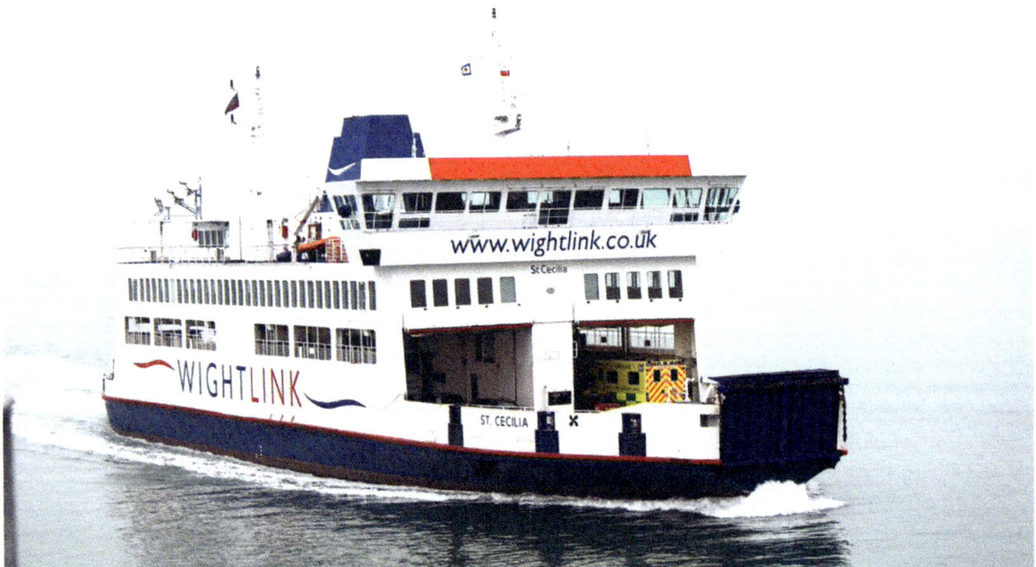

Yet again the Isle of Wight vehicle was to surface unexpectedly, but this time nearer its home base. It is pictured on car ferry *St Cecilia* approaching Portsmouth Harbour from the island. 5 September 2014.

Motorcycle Response Unit (MRU)

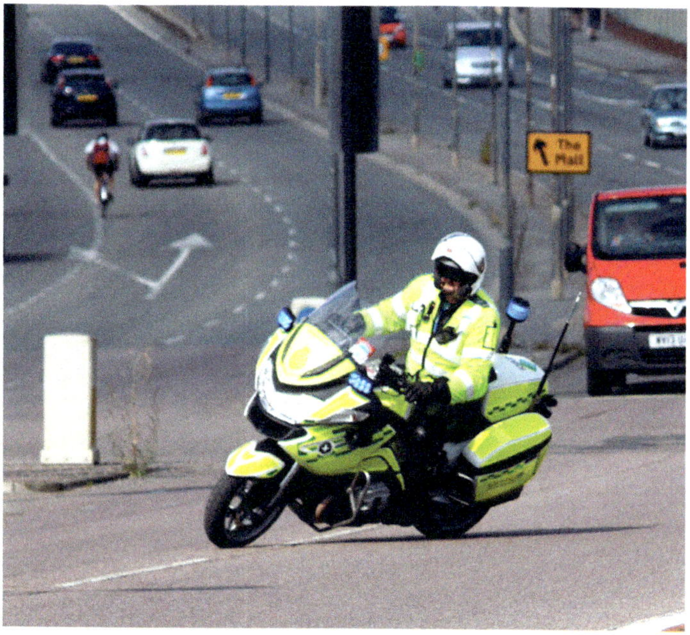

This SWASFT unit is able to deploy as a group, such as with three or four machines, anywhere within the region for a specific task (such as a major event with large crowds due) or to operate individually. 10 September 2014.

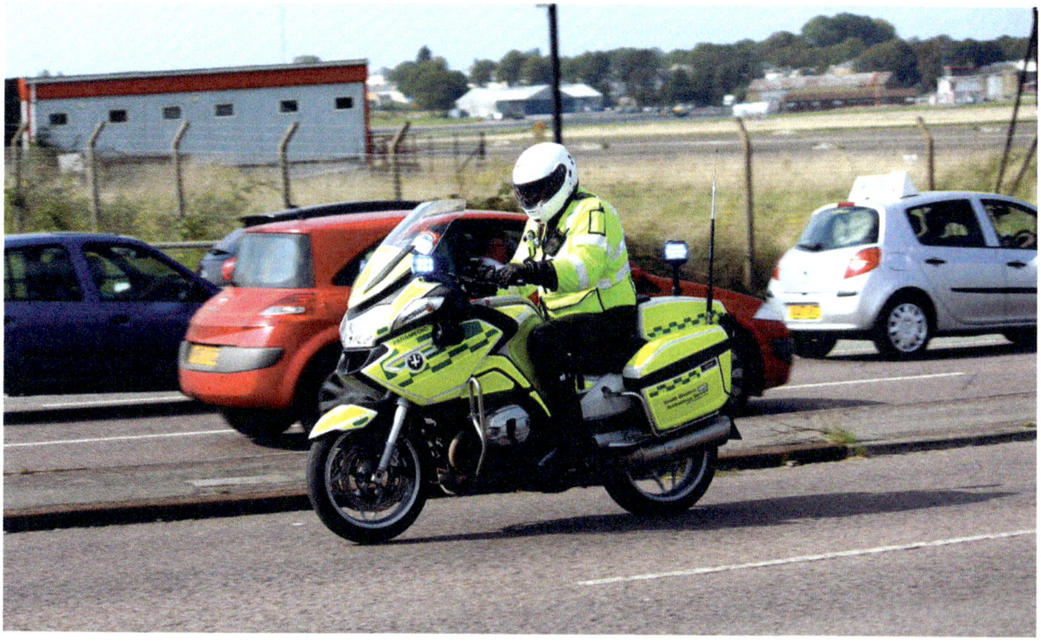

LJ13 FPF was static when seen on the A38 inbound carriageway at Filton, with the Tour of Britain cycle race due any minute. However, an emergency call saw its hurried departure. In the distant background are the former police and air ambulance bases, pictured prior to the excellent new Concorde Museum being built in 2017 and the bases moving to Almondsbury during the latter part of 2018. 10 September 2014.

NHS Blood and Transplant/Blood Bikes

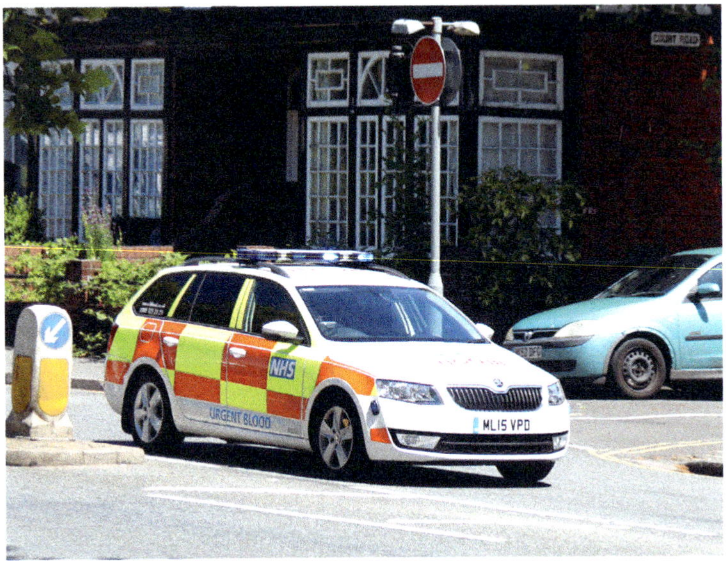
NHS
URGENT BLOOD
ML15 VPD

Based at the NHS Blood & Transplant (NHSBT) blood-processing complex at North Bristol Park, Filton, this Skoda estate is regularly observed heading in and out of Bristol. Seeing it on the blues and twos is, however, far less common. The Filton blood-processing complex is reputedly the world's biggest. 2 July 2017.

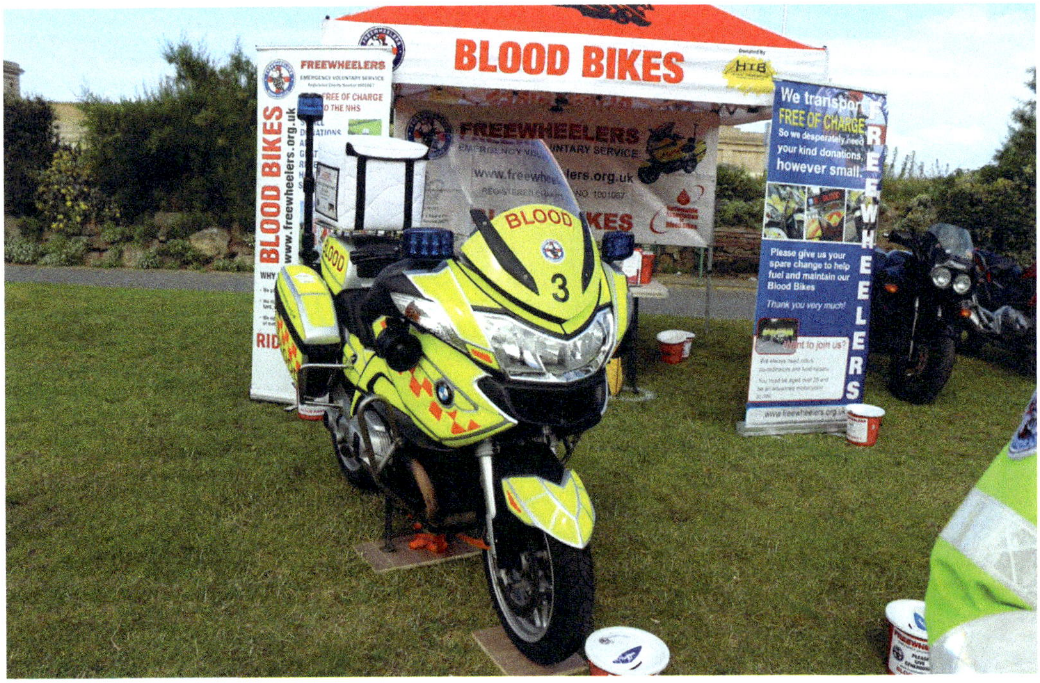
BLOOD BIKES
FREEWHEELERS
BLOOD BIKES
www.freewheelers.org.uk
FREEWHEELERS
EMERGENCY VOLUNTARY SERVICE
BLOOD
3
We transport
FREE OF CHARGE
So we desperately need your kind donations,
however small.
FREEWHEELERS
Please give us your spare change to help fuel and maintain our Blood Bikes
Thank you very much!

Sterling work is undertaken on a purely voluntary basis by the Freewheelers organisation (otherwise known as Blood Bikes), who ferry blood, breast milk and other medical supplies as required among hospitals and make daily deliveries to air ambulance bases in South Gloucestershire and Wiltshire. Much of this work is undertaken on call during the evening, night and weekends. Strategically placed buckets at this Weston-super-Mare display hopefully encouraged the public to financially donate to this very worthy cause. 3 July 2016.

Patient Transport Service

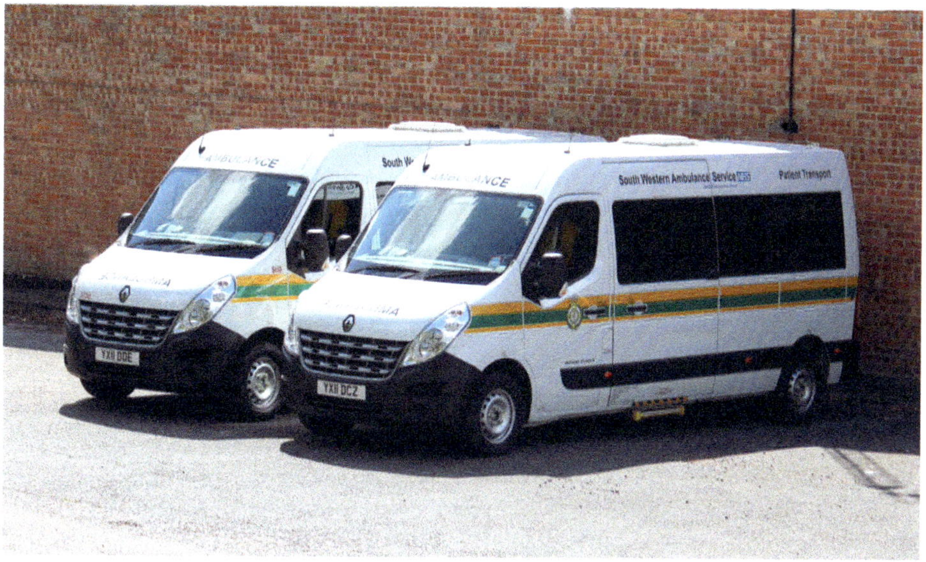

Prior to repainting in large all-over blocks of green and yellow battenburg livery, this pair of Patient Transport Service units are pictured out of service at the side of the former Tower Hill central ambulance station, Bristol. 9 August 2014.

Rapid Response Vehicles (RRV)

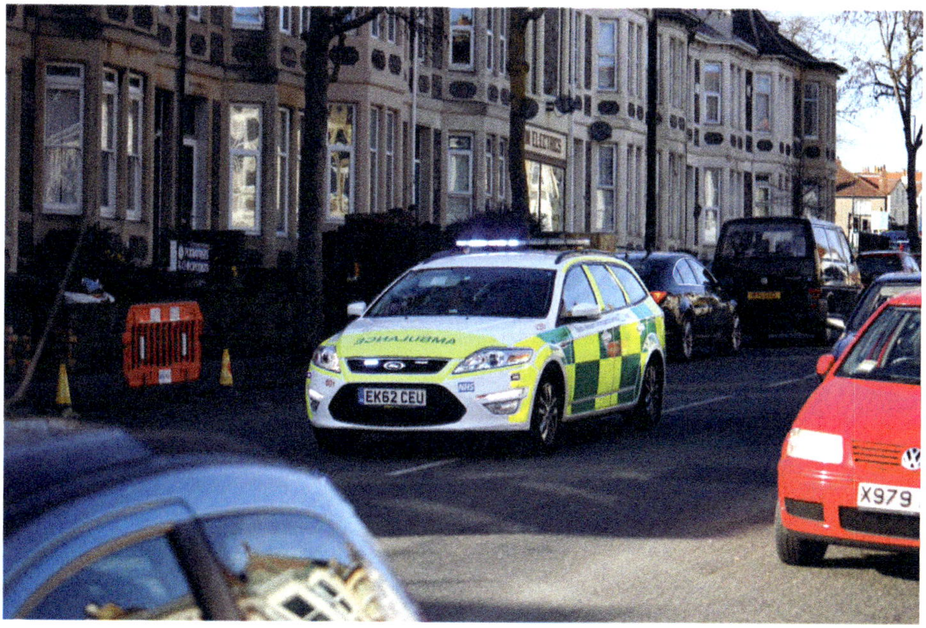

Ford Mondeo estate EK62 CEU is pictured at speed responding from Horfield Common towards central Bristol on an emergency. 13 March 2015.

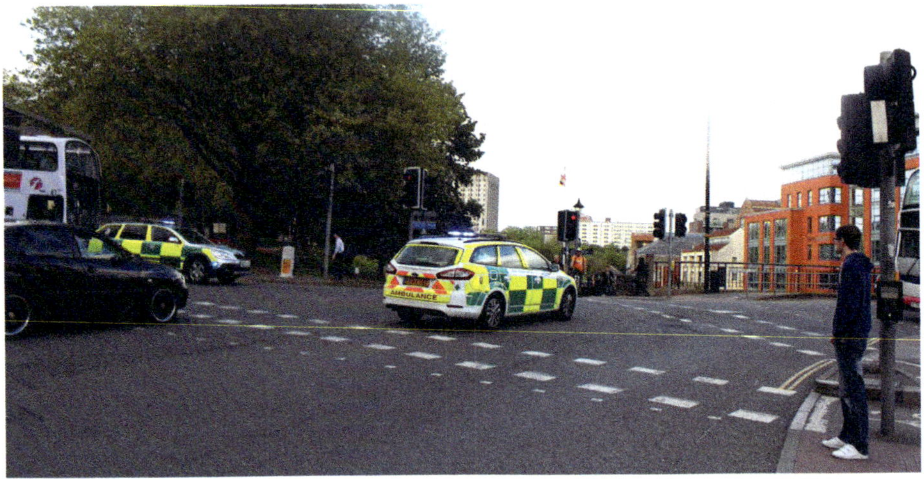

The critical moment as both RRVs on the blues on separate emergency calls, sirens blaring, need to simultaneously negotiate the same junction while going in opposing directions! WF13 YJR, the Skoda vehicle on the left, needs to turn to its right towards the camera position to go down Baldwin Street while Ford Mondeo EK62 CDF, having come up Baldwin Street, is turning right to go across Bristol Bridge. The skill of both drivers, in always being mindful of meeting a fellow emergency vehicle on the blues at a blind junction, whereby neither vehicle was visible to the other until the very last moment, avoided the conflict that could so easily have resulted in disastrous consequences. 15 May 2014.

St John Ambulance (SJA)

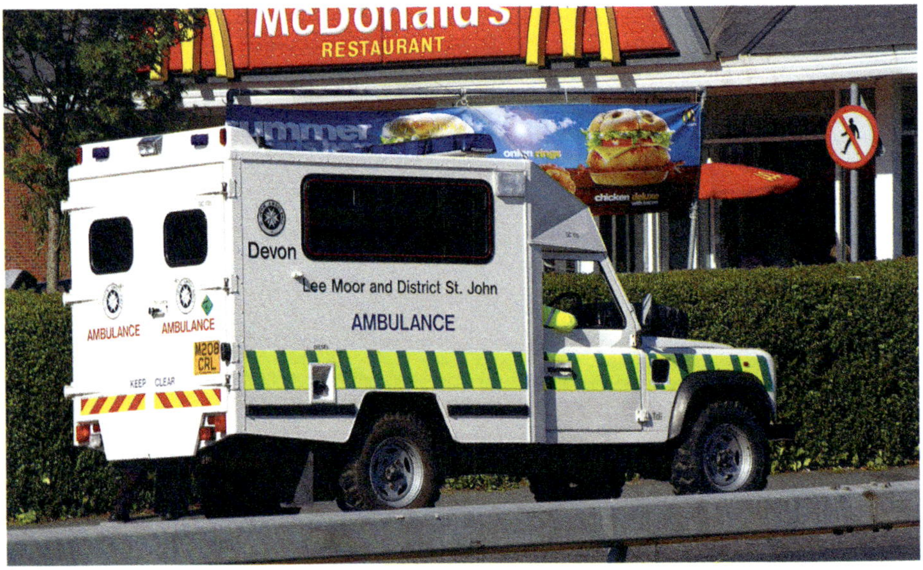

Land Rover M208 CRL heads from Plympton towards the Marsh Mills roundabout, Plymouth. Like the British Red Cross, SJA are a largely volunteer organisation devoting a great deal of their time to training and providing first aid cover at numerous public events up and down the land. 14 July 2006.

Chapter 2

Coastal and Inland Waterway Rescue Services

The sea respects no one; fortunately, the emergency services are only too aware of its dangers and, accordingly, the resources they can muster on a full-time or voluntary basis to the open sea or inland waterways are considerable. This chapter provides a selection of that vast response in the West of England. Included is a glimpse into neighbouring Hampshire with emergency responses typical of those to be found in the West of England. For emergencies at sea dial '999' and ask for the coastguard.

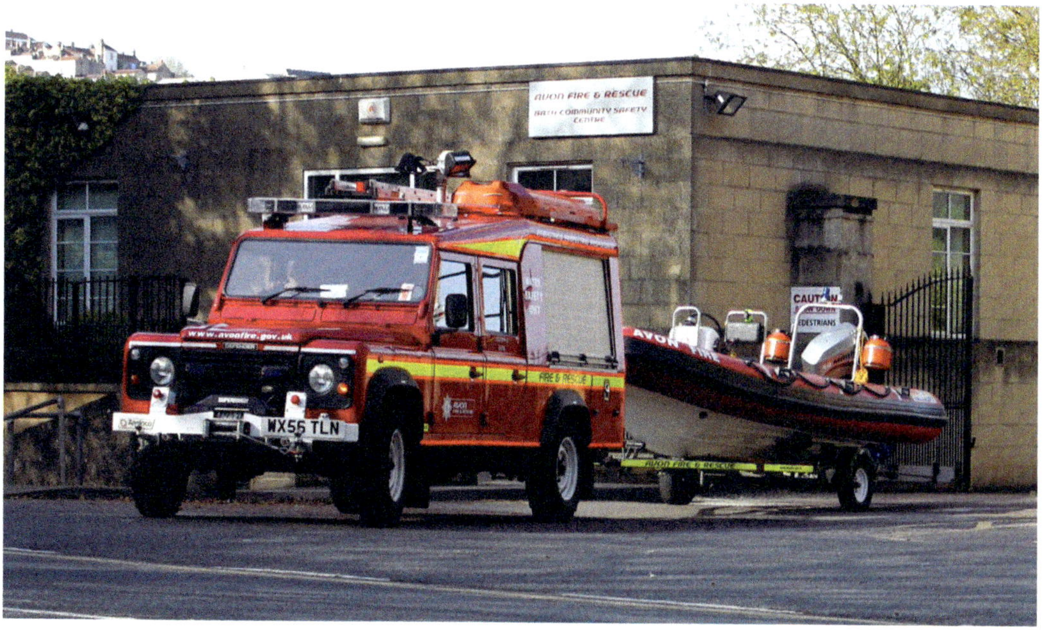

This 2012 image shows Bath's Water Safety Unit, comprising a Land Rover Defender 130, registration WX56 TLN, towing a Valiant RIB (Rigid Inflatable Boat). A Mercedes Sprinter Rescue Boat Unit went on the run at Bath in late 2018.

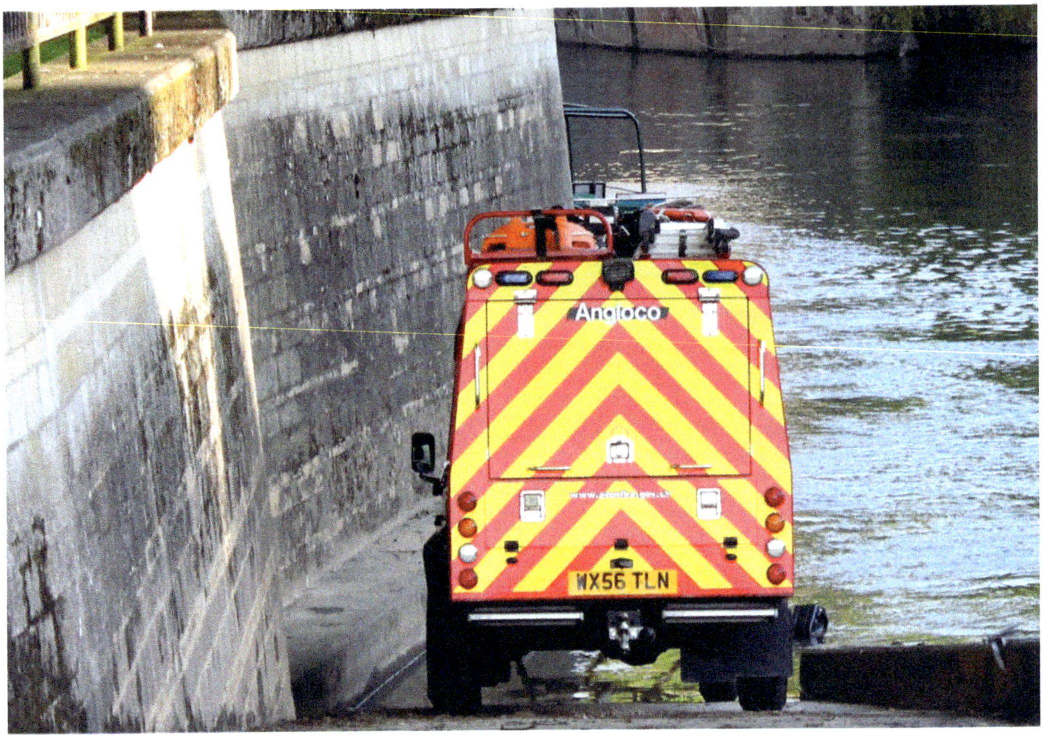

The brigade has a dedicated slipway for launch purposes at the junction of Ferry Lane and Spring Gardens Road, Bath. The boat trailer is affixed to the front of the Land Rover, which then drives slowly down the ramp. 2012.

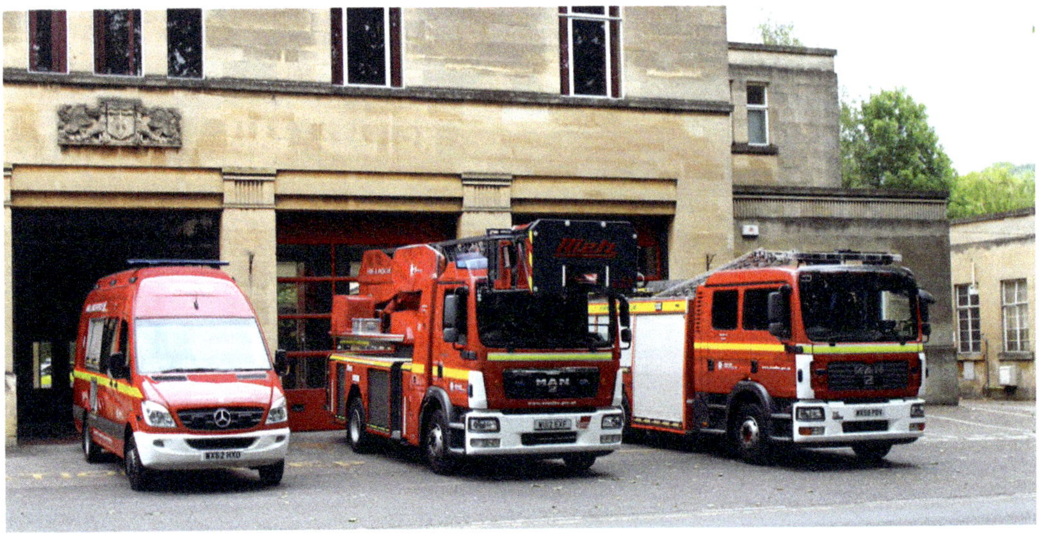

Also on the run at Bath is a Mercedes Animal/Water Rescue Unit with a counterpart on the run at Bedminster, Bristol. Bath's A/WRU, WX62 HXO, is pictured alongside the station's turntable ladder and retained crew water tender ladder, registrations WU12 EXF and WX58 PDV respectively. 20 June 2015.

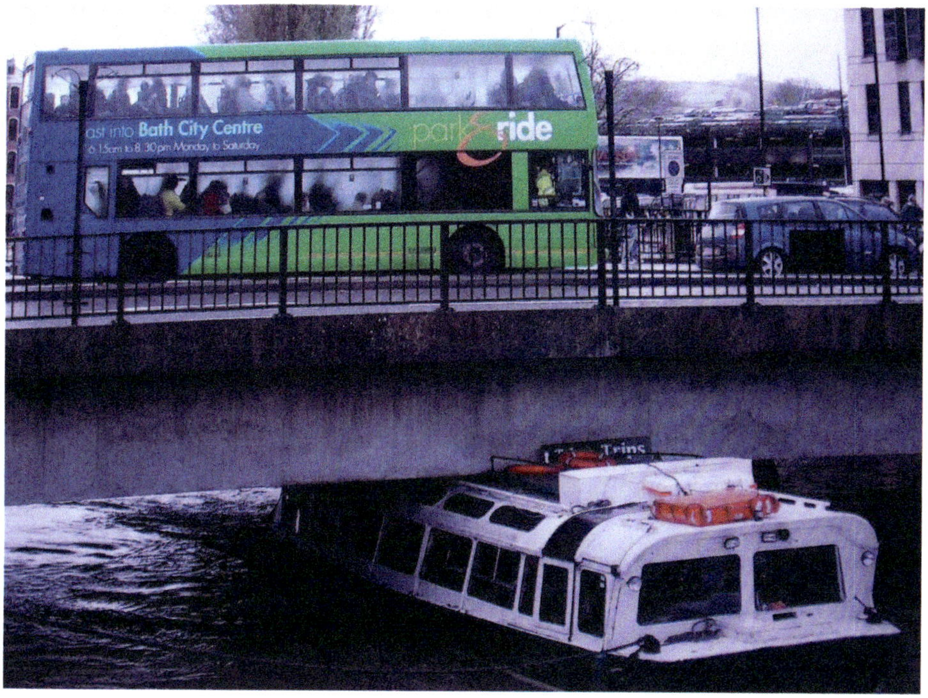

The power of floodwater resulted in a Bath pleasure boat breaking free of its moorings near Pulteney Bridge and lodging some 700 metres downstream under Churchill Bridge. Fortunately no one was aboard the vessel at the time. Early 2000s.

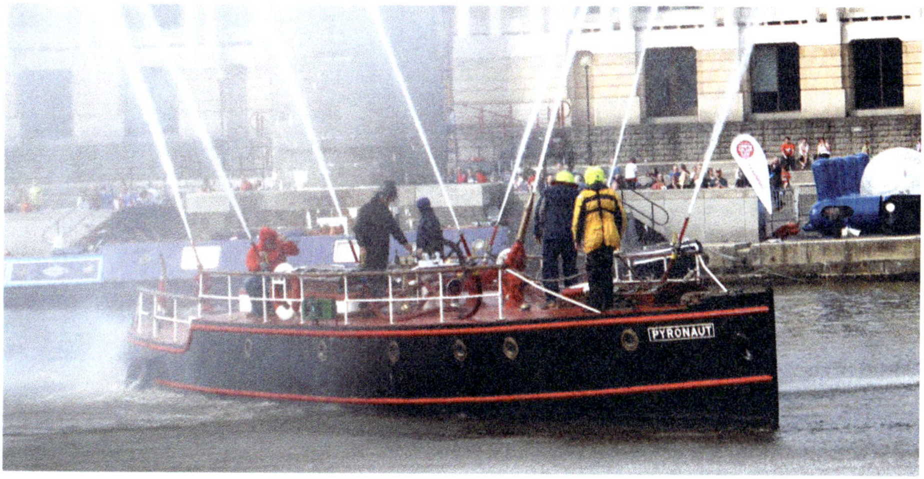

Fires in property adjoining waterways have seen brigades with fireboats respond. Former Bristol Fire Brigade fireboat *Pyronaut* is preserved in the city docks, where it is seen demonstrating its immense power by firing eight jets into the air – the roar of its mighty engines is a sound never to be forgotten! It sailed on the evening tide from Bristol Docks to supplement fireboat *Endres* Gane, which was stationed in the Avonmouth Docks at the massive sixty-pump oil refinery fire that broke out on the afternoon of 6 September 1951. Supporting appliances came from as far as Plymouth. 2010.

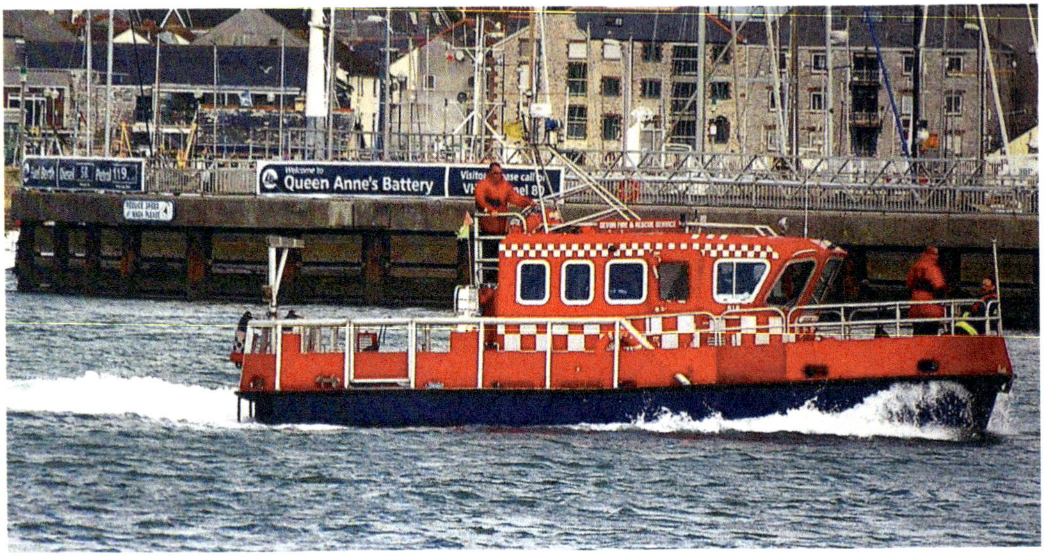

The Devon Fire & Rescue Service boat *Vigilis* (pictured prior to amalgamation with Somerset, which occurred on 1 April 2007) is seen returning to its Turnchapel moorings, Plymouth. 2005.

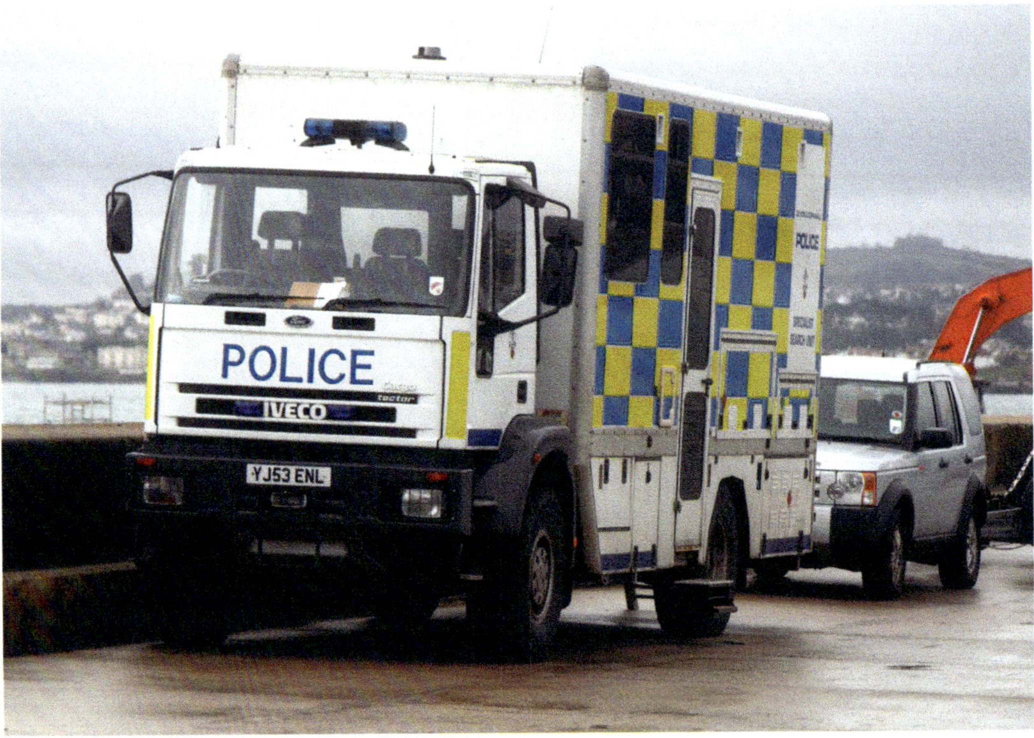

The Devon & Cornwall Police Ford Iveco specialist search unit YJ53 ENL is seen parked on Torquay Harbour as its divers search for a possible murder weapon. This vehicle was originally in use with North Yorkshire Police. 2010.

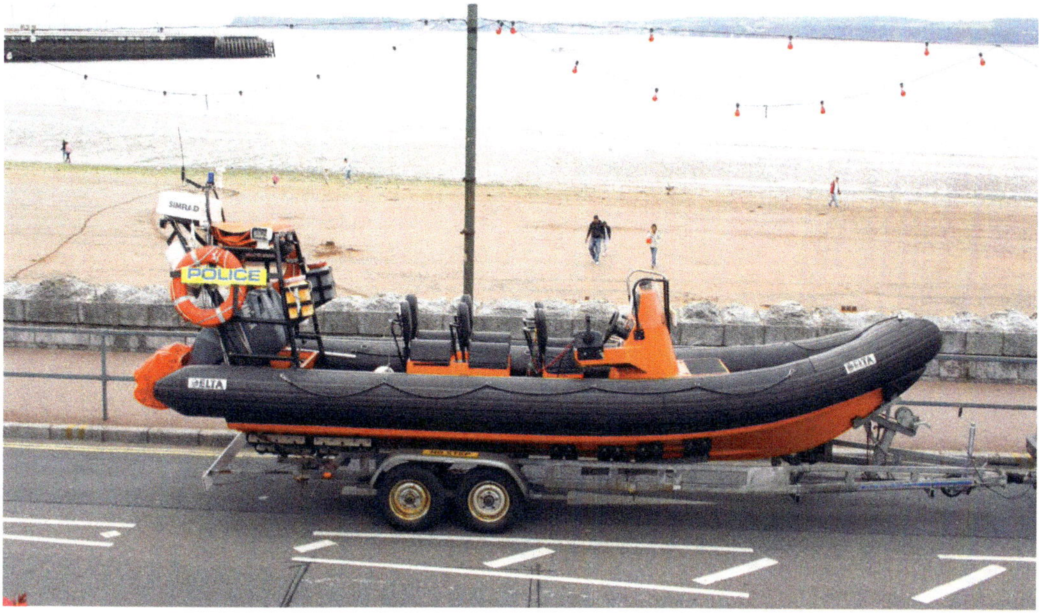

The Devon & Cornwall Police rigid inflatable boat being towed along Torquay seafront. 2010.

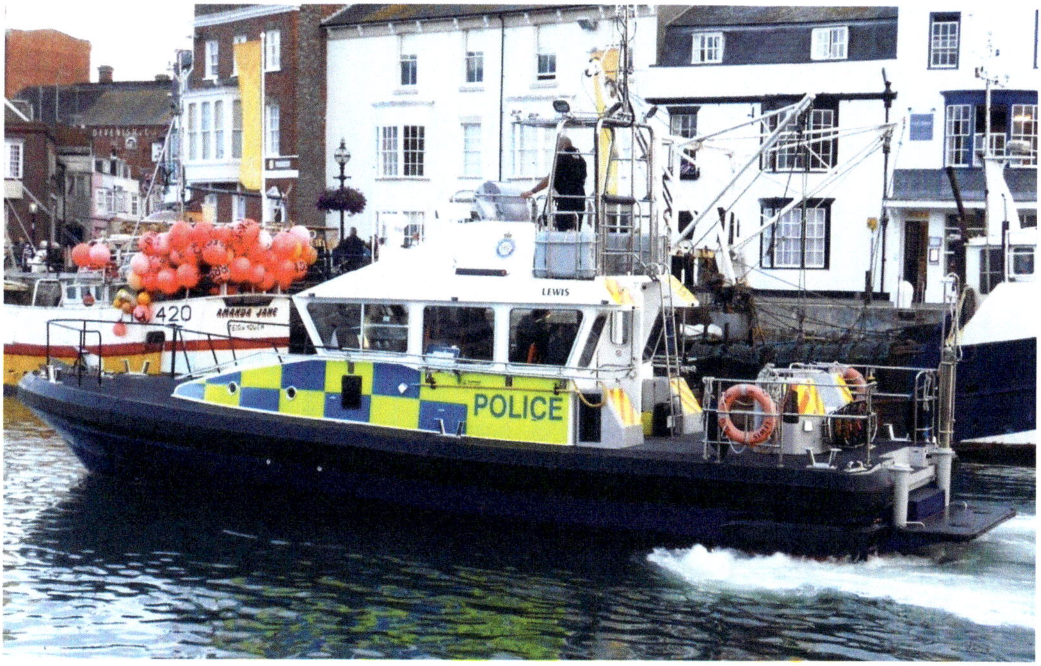

New Ministry of Defence Police launch *Lewis*, pictured in Weymouth for the waterborne section of the 2012 summer Olympics. Many of the force's new craft serve at Faslane, Scotland, hence their naming after Scottish islands. Summer 2012. (Image: Matt Holmes)

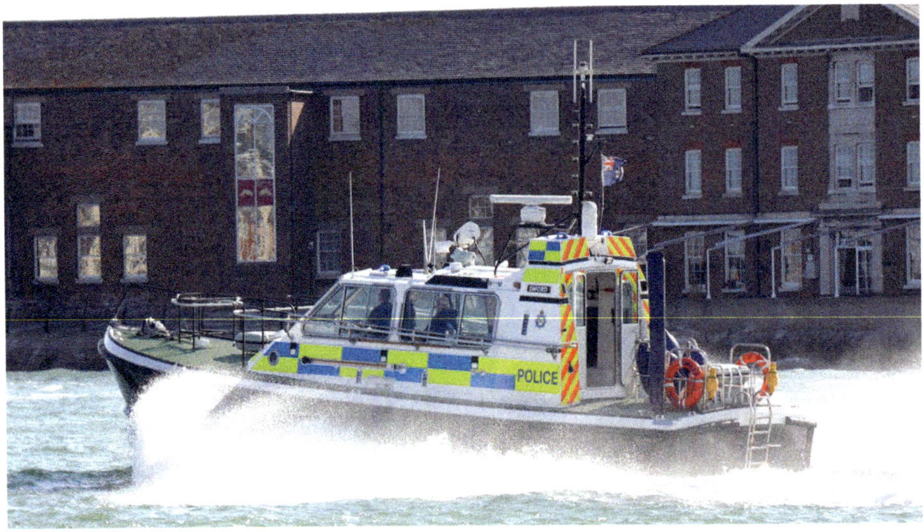

Ministry of Defence Police launches – identical to Portsmouth's launch *Sword*, pictured above on the blue light at high speed thrashing the waves as it responds to a yacht in distress in the Solent – patrol the waters surrounding HM Naval Base, Devonport, Plymouth. 2011.

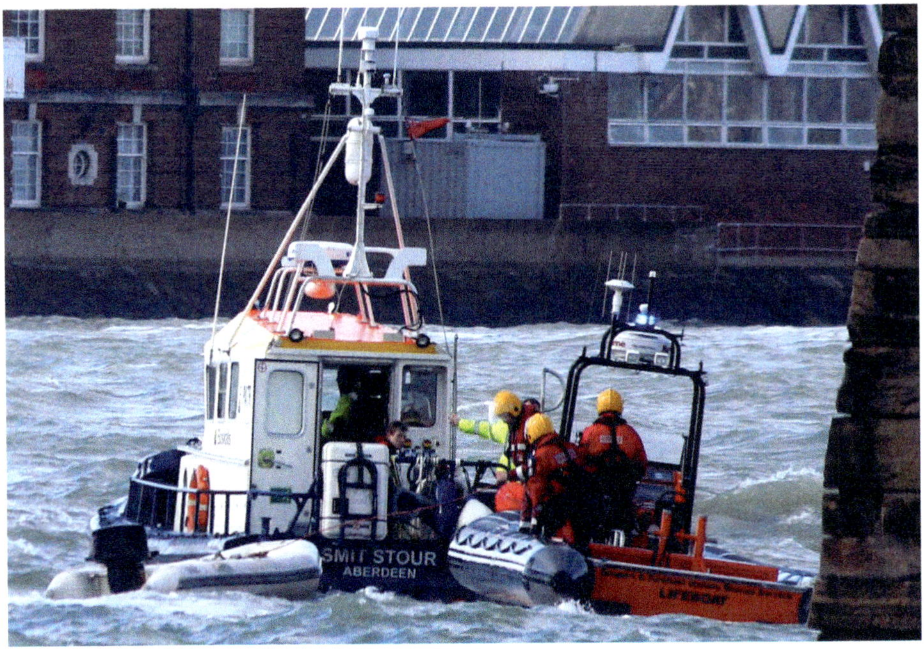

This image, also taken at the entrance to Portsmouth Harbour, shows the dangerous waters where youths have just been rescued from their flimsy dinghy during Storm Katie and taken onboard the vessel *Smit Stour*. The volunteer Gosport & Fareham Inshore Rescue Service lifeboat arrived moments later and its crew are in the process of securing the dinghy. Deep, swirling waters such as these can be found along the extensive coastline of the West of England counties. 27 March 2016.

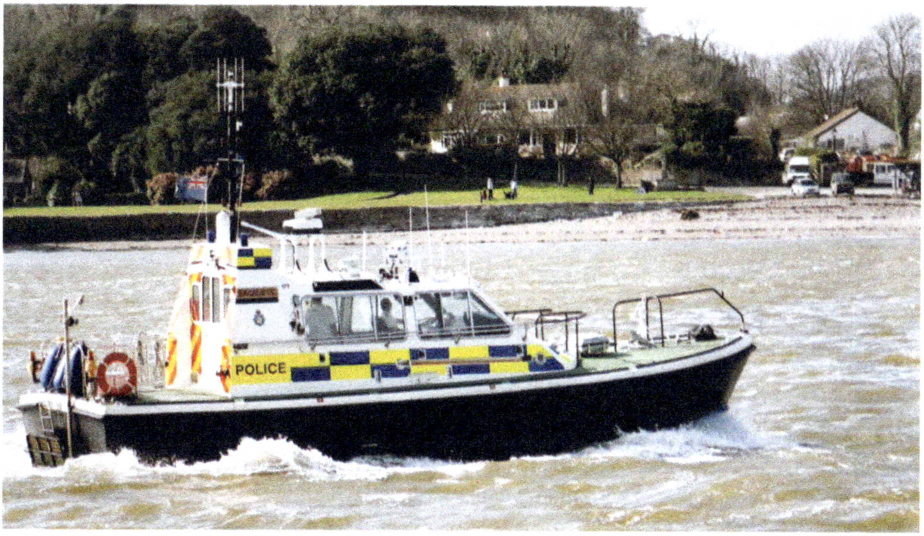

The River Tamar, marking the boundary between Devon and Cornwall, leads out into Plymouth Sound and is the route used by naval vessels, the larger ones under MOD Police launch escort as they enter and leave their base. *Excalibur* is pictured returning to Devonport naval base from such an escort, with the Cornish coast visible in the background. These waters off Devil's Point hide treacherous currents just below the surface. 2006.

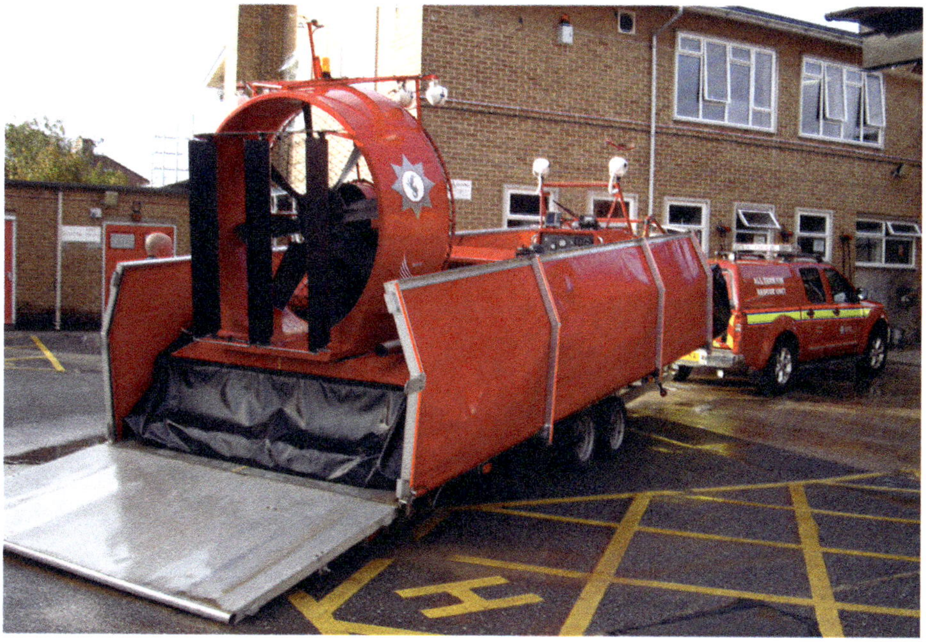

Avon FRS Hovercraft on its temporary trailer before the retired Bath turntable ladder Y561 XAE was converted in 2011 to carry the versatile craft based at Weston-super-Mare. The tide in the Bristol Channel has the second highest rise and fall in the world, stranding many a visitor a long way offshore at low tide when the tide turns and rapidly races over the mud banks. 24 October 2009. (Image: James Roberts)

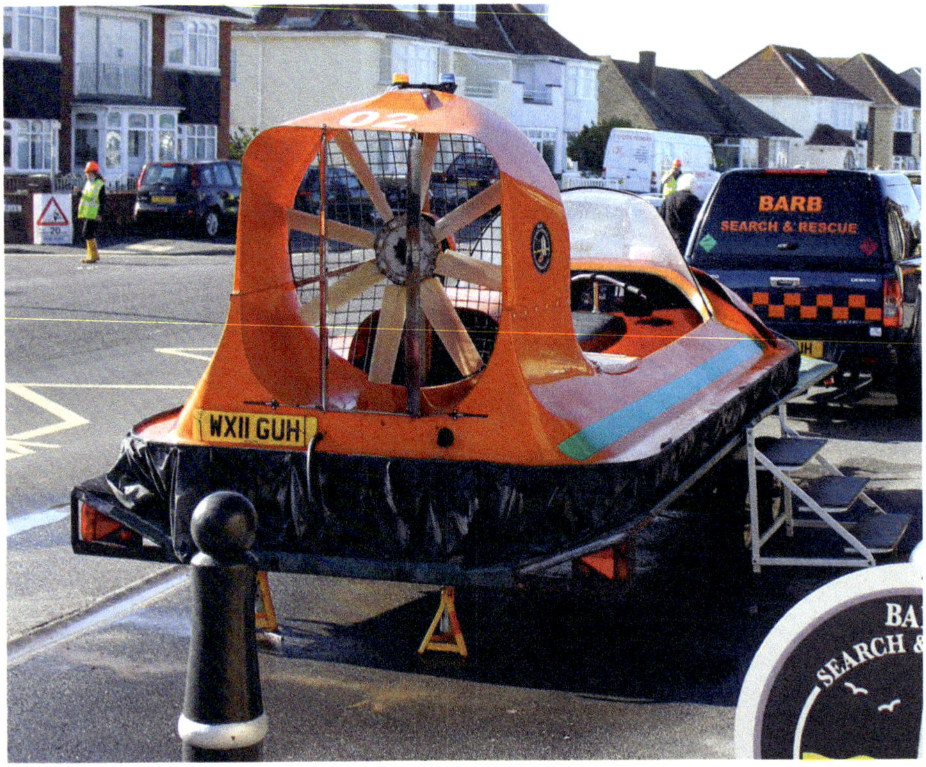

The Burnham Area Rescue Boat (BARB), one of two regularly deployed hovercraft stationed at Burnham-on-Sea and operated by the volunteers helping protect the coastline. 31 August 2014.

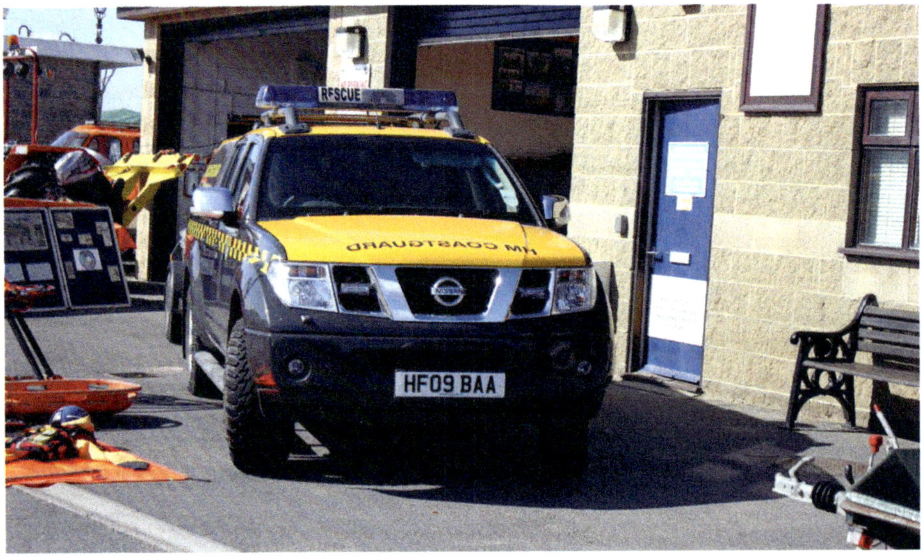

HM Coastguard, Burnham-on-Sea, co-located with BARB on the seafront in the centre of the town. The RNLI base is nearby. 31 August 2014.

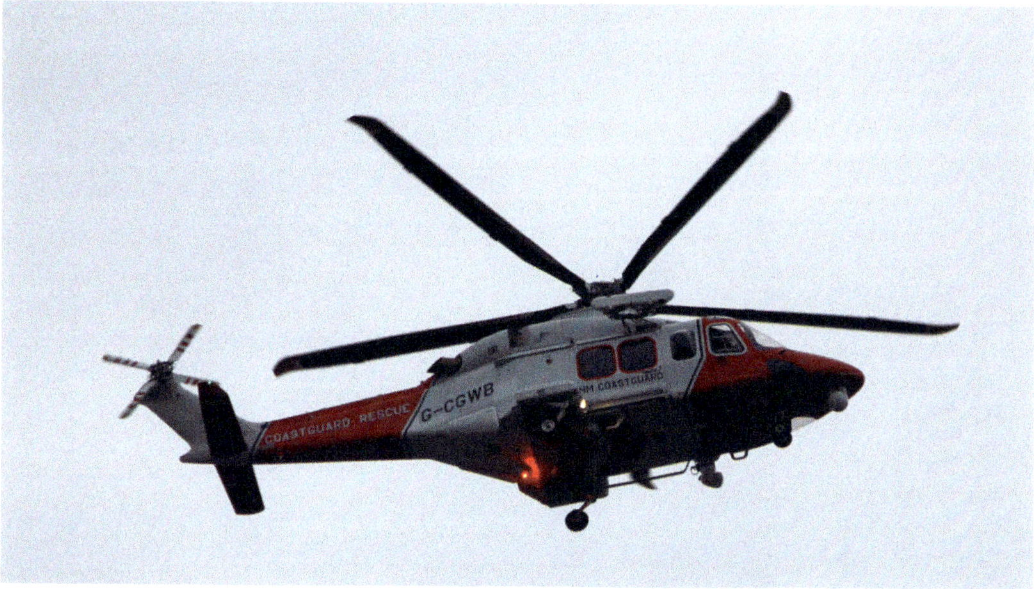

Heading over Bristol in light drizzle on a reconnaissance flight to view the helipads at the Bristol Royal Infirmary and Southmead Hospital is HM Coastguard's all-weather AW169, call sign Rescue 106, registration G-CGWB, which was then based at Portland, Dorset. 18 August 2014.

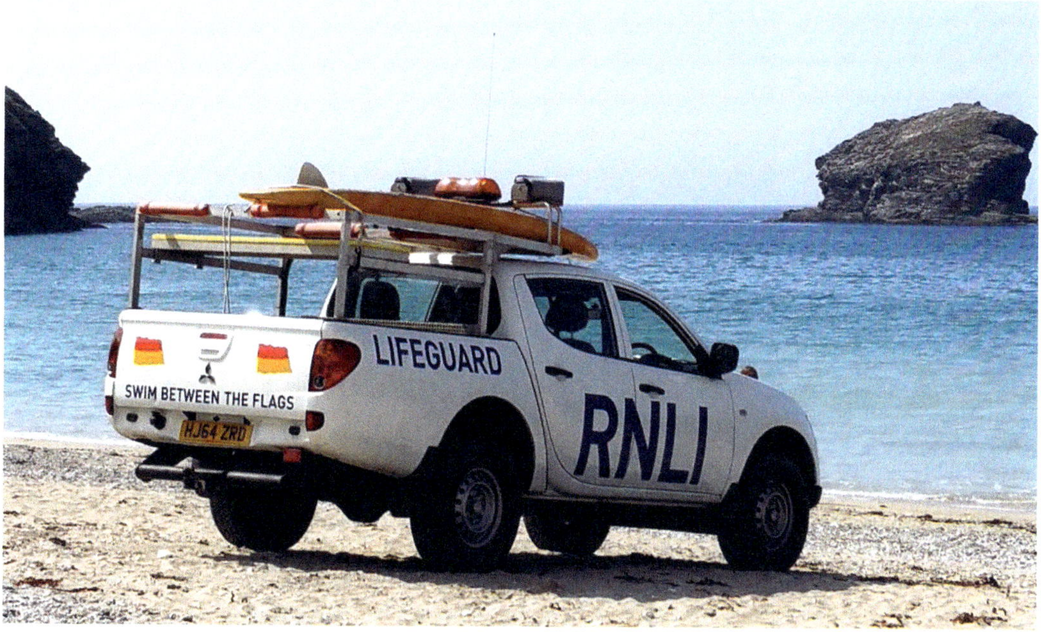

This type of vehicle is a typical summer sight, and is used in this example by RNLI lifeguards as they help keep everyone safe on the beach at Portreath. Thanks to an observant RNLI lifeguard, 15 miles further up the Cornish coast two children aged six and twelve on holiday from Glasgow were rescued in the late July 2018 heatwave, having strayed into deep water at Crantock, near Newquay. May 2016. (Image: Matt Holmes)

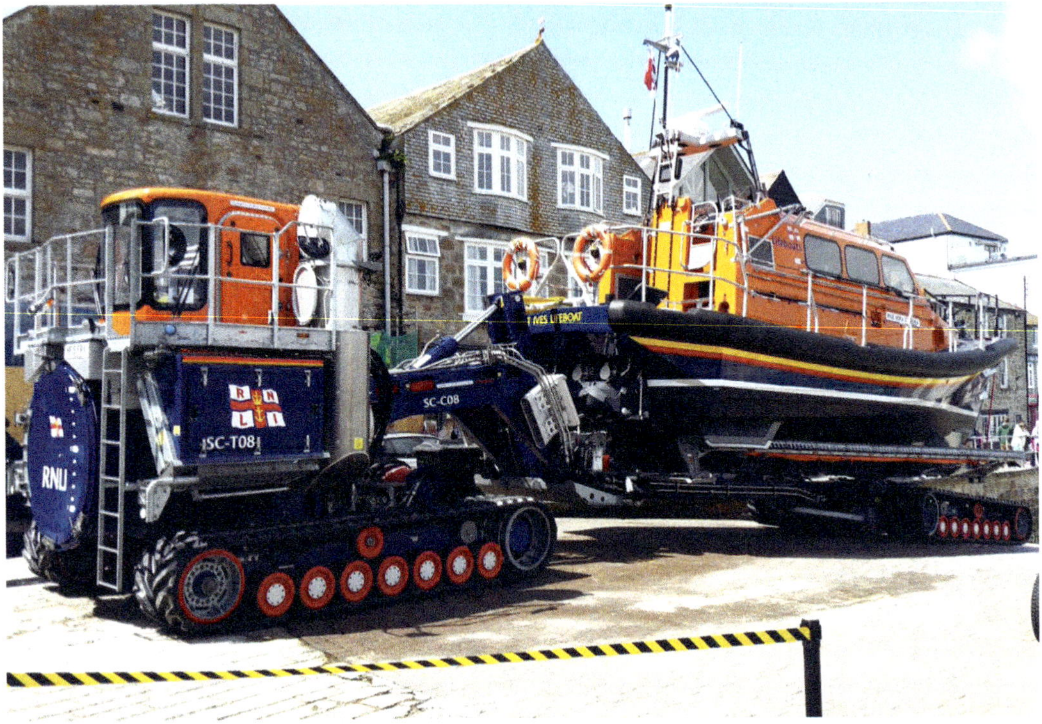

The St Ives lifeboat being trundled into position for an exercise launch. May 2016. (Image: Matt Holmes)

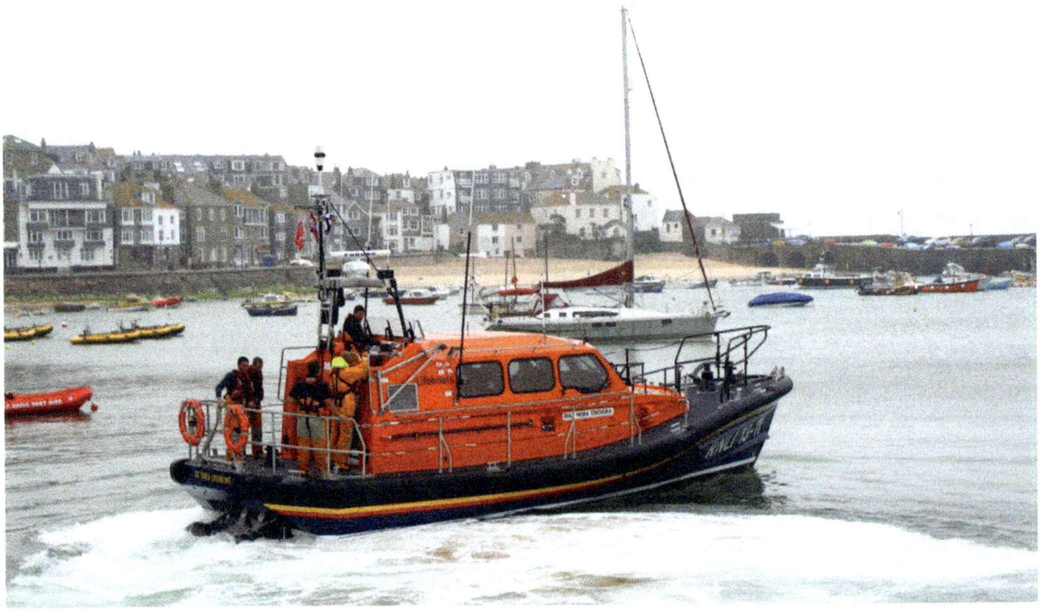

The station operates a 2015 all-weather Shannon class vessel, 13-11 *Nora Stachura,* and D-803, an inshore rescue boat. May 2016. (Image: Matt Holmes)

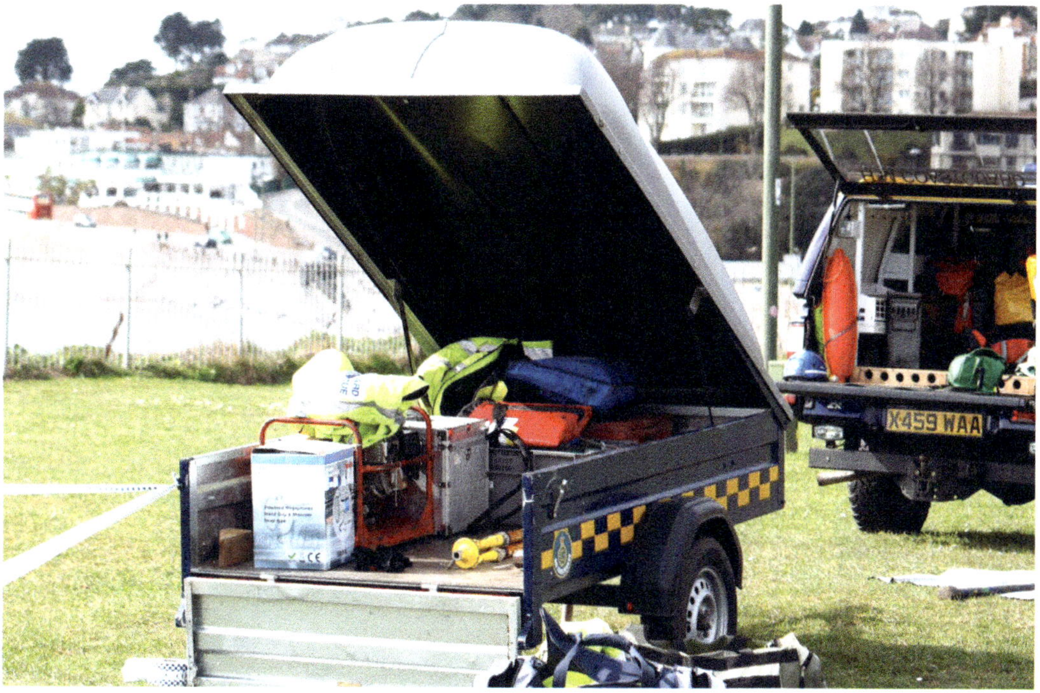

A HM Coastguard vehicle and trailer positioned for an exercise with the RNLI at Corbyn Head, Torquay. 2010.

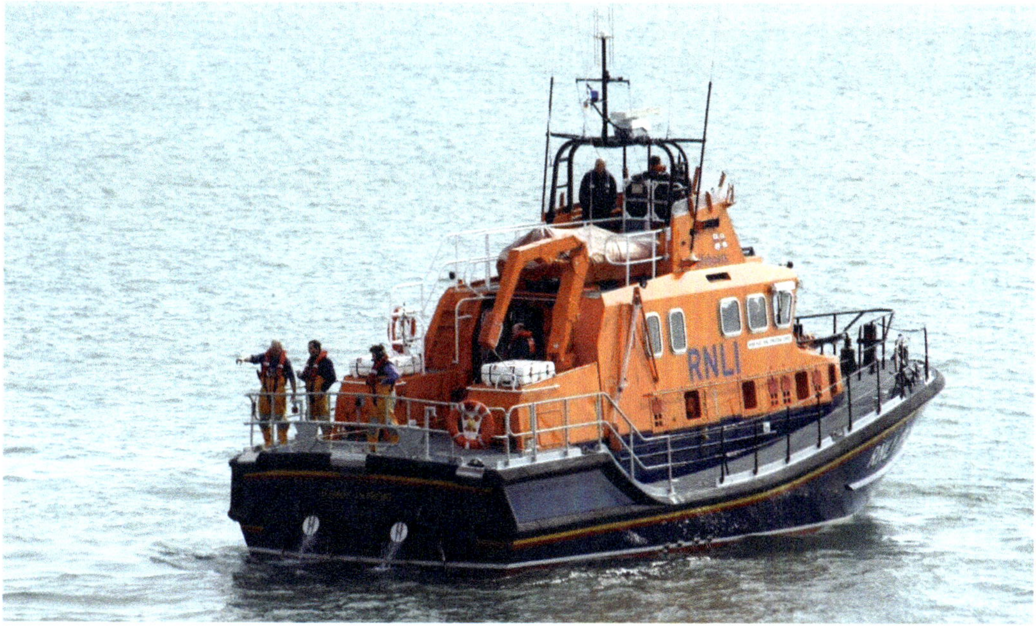

The 2001 RNLI Severn class Torbay all-weather lifeboat 17-28 *Alec and Christina Dykes* remains offshore during this exercise as its inshore rescue boat deploys at the base of the cliff. A 'casualty' will be winched up the cliff to the waiting HM Coastguard personnel.

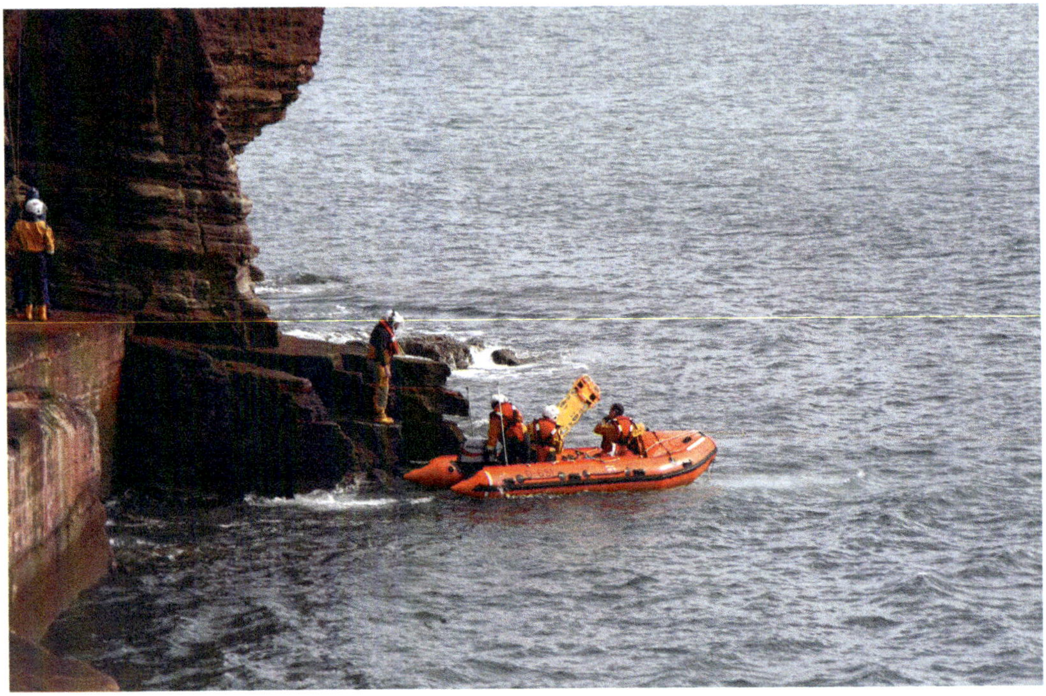

D-651, the Torbay-based inshore rescue boat, manoeuvres at the base of cliffs at Corbyn Head in order for the crew to pass a spinal board to colleagues.

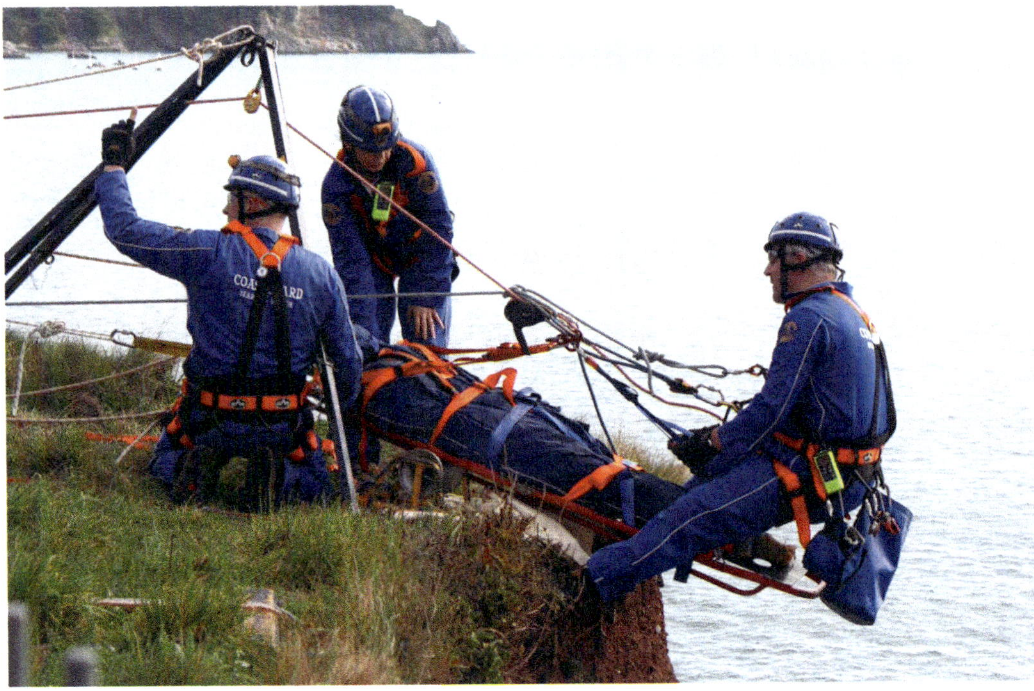

With the 'casualty' safely up on the headland, the exercise draws to a close. 2010.

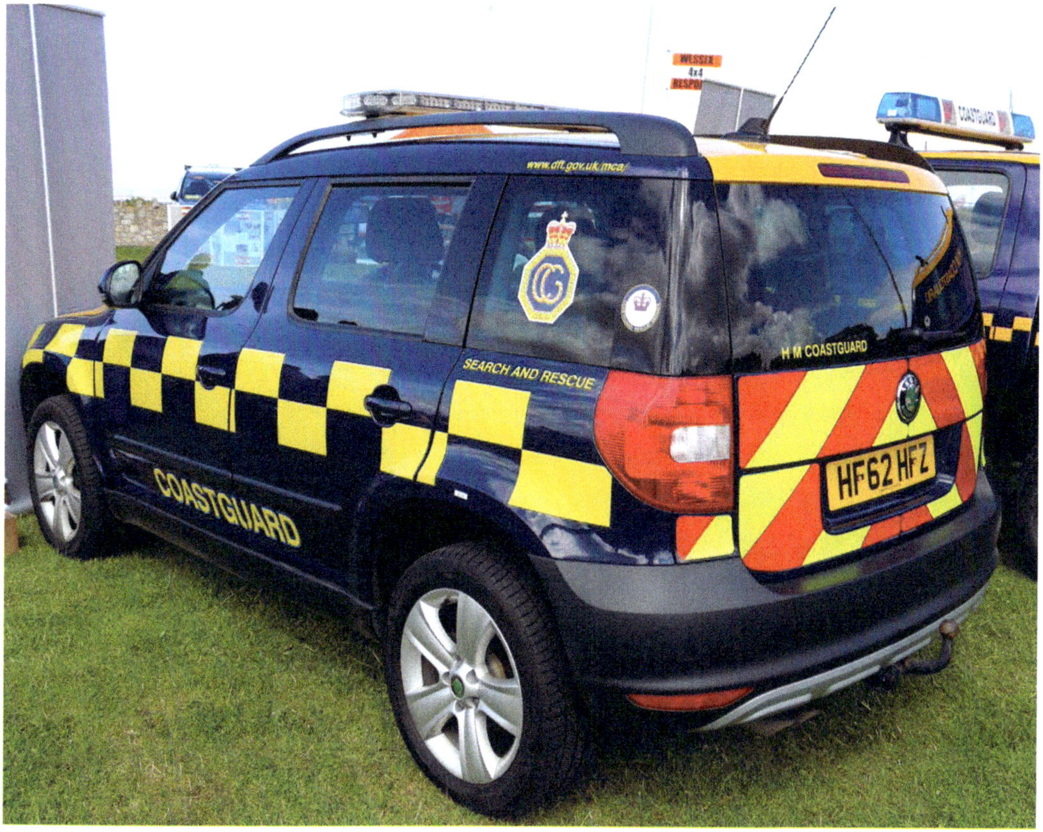

A modern Skoda HM Coastguard vehicle, HF62 HFZ, is pictured on the Beach Lawns at one of the excellent Weston-super-Mare lifeboat days. 3 July 2016.

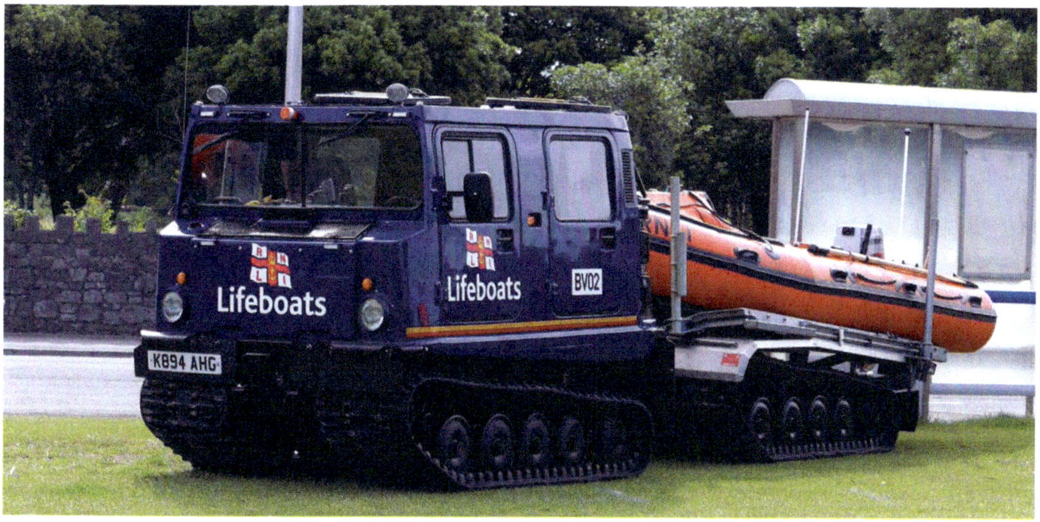

Weston-super-Mare's two RNLI craft on display that day were the larger Atlantic 75 class B-769 *Coventry & Warwickshire* and (above) D-735, the inshore rescue boat. 3 July 2016.

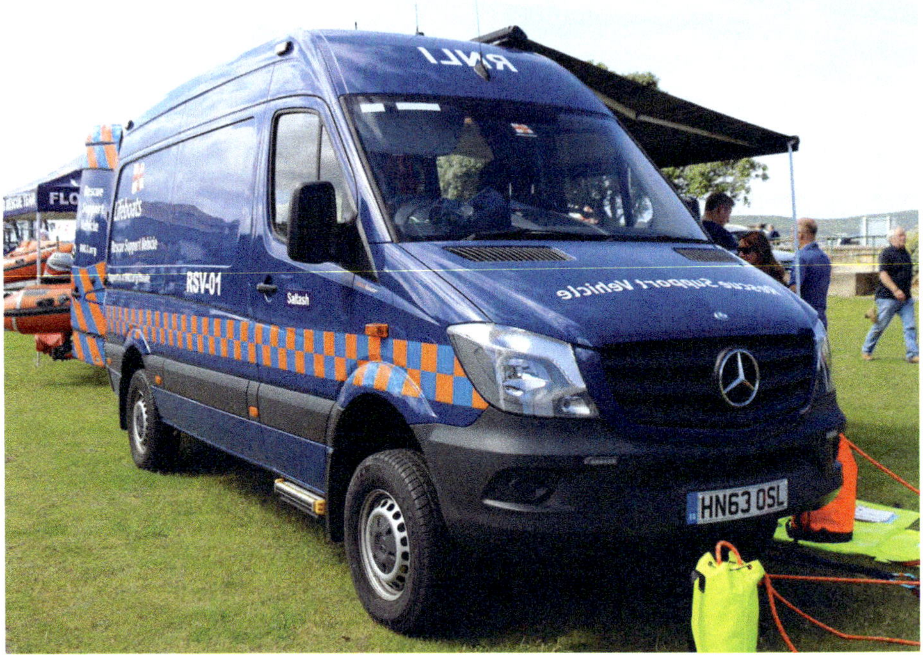

RNLI Mercedes Rescue Support Vehicle RSV-01, registration HN63 OSL, which was based at Saltash, Cornwall, also made a very welcome appearance at the Weston-super-Mare event. 3 July 2016.

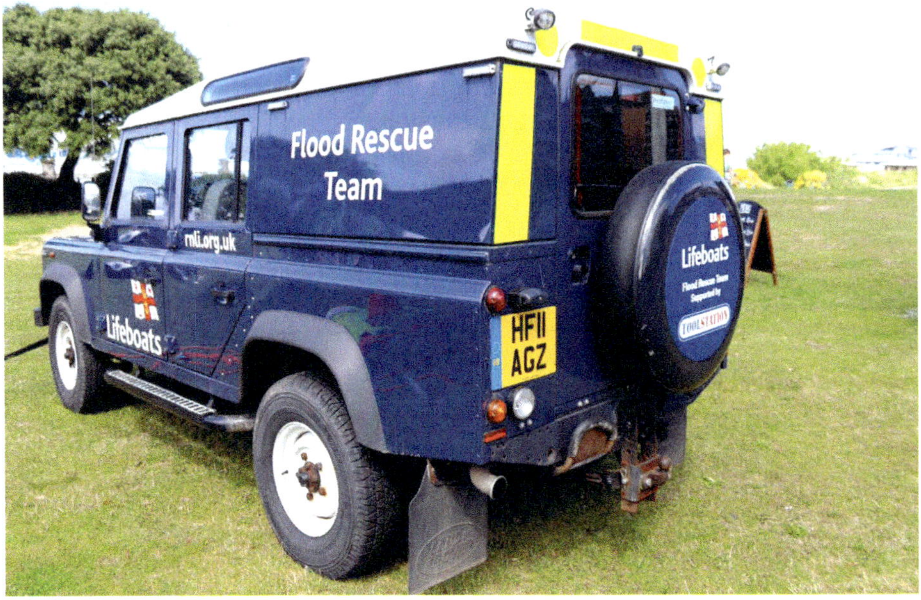

Another rare sighting on the same date was Land Rover Flood Rescue Team vehicle HF11 AGZ. 3 July 2016.

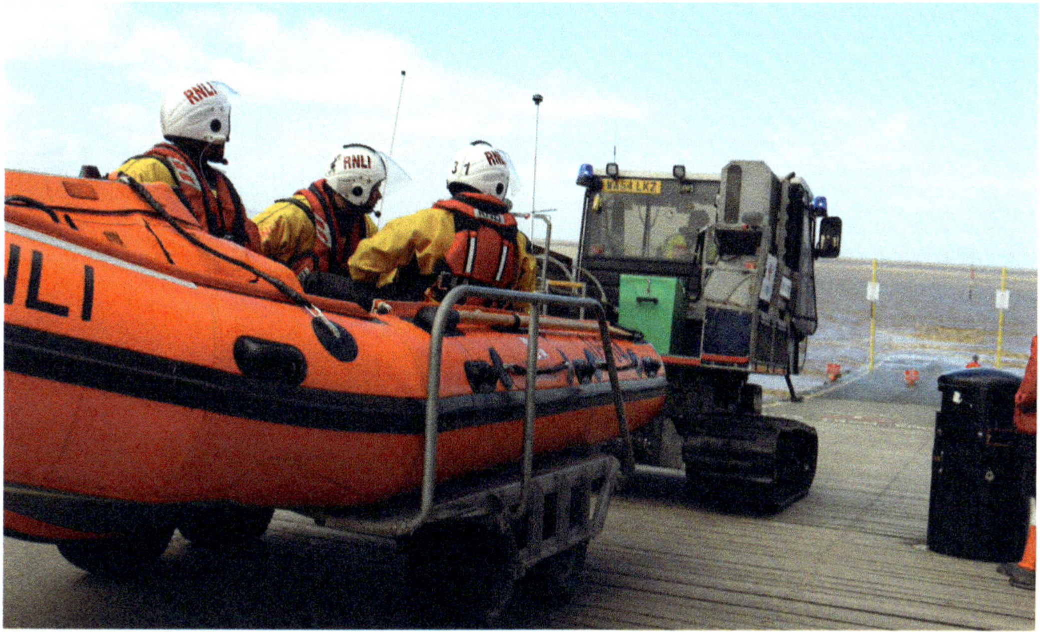

At Burnham-on-Sea the annual 999 display is a well attended event. The year 2016 was to be no exception, with both of the town's lifeboats being launched in a simulated emergency. Burnham-on-Sea's RNLI station is set back a short distance from the seafront launch ramp. As a result its inshore rescue boats are towed in purpose-built cradles with the crew already dressed and onboard. The D-class lifeboat heads for the water. 7 August 2016.

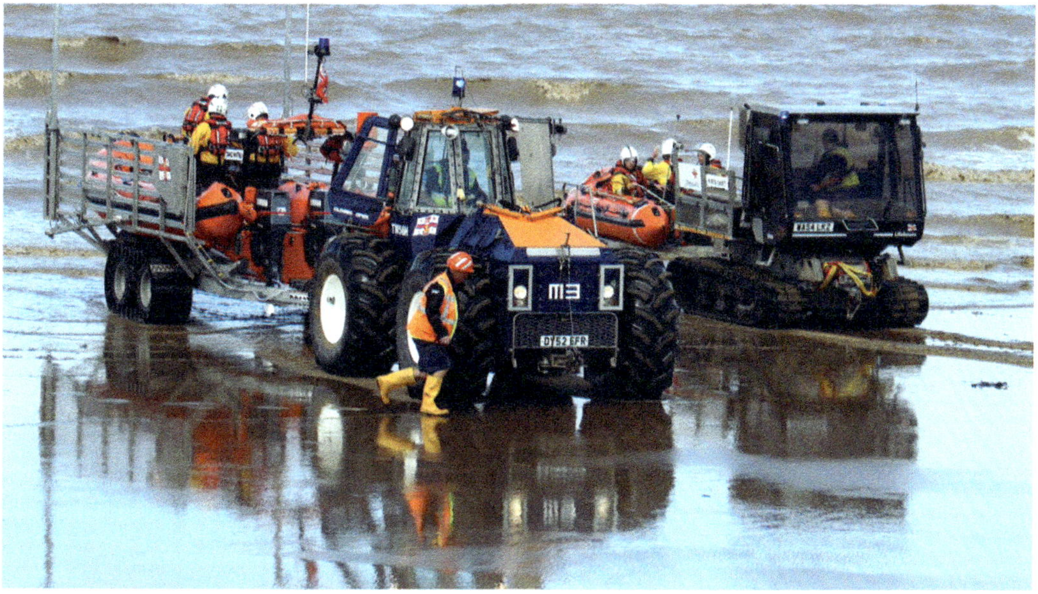

Both towing units are pictured as under the direction of a launchmaster they prepare to launch their lifeboats.The towing units reverse into the water, thus enabling the rescue boats to float free from their cradles and literally hit the waves with their engines already running. 7 August 2016.

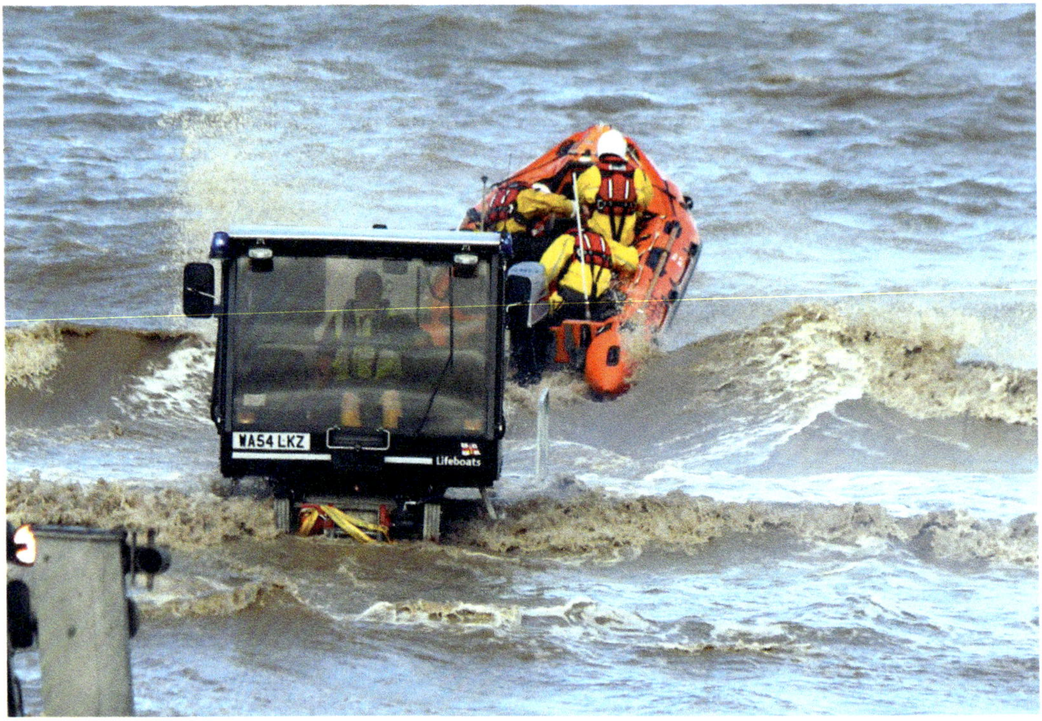

D-664 leaps out of its cradle, its single outboard motor slicing through the waves. 7 August 2016.

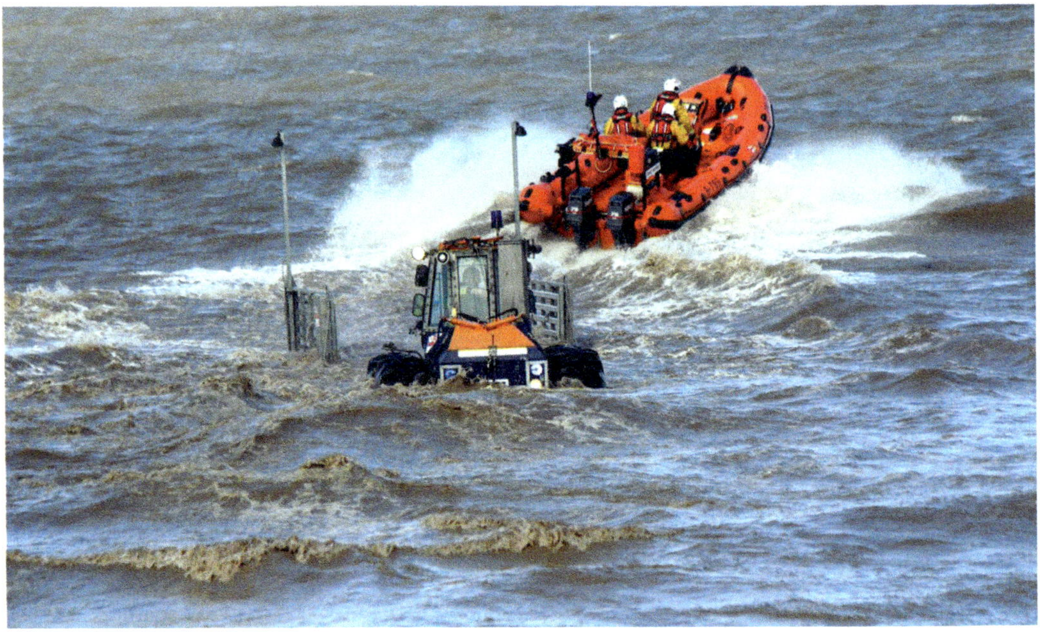

The RNLI's 2004 B-class Atlantic 75 inshore lifeboat B-795 *Staines Whitfield* is buoyant, the tyres of the tractor unit now almost submerged. Both outboard motors dig into the waves, rapidly propelling the craft on its 'mission'. 7 August 2016.

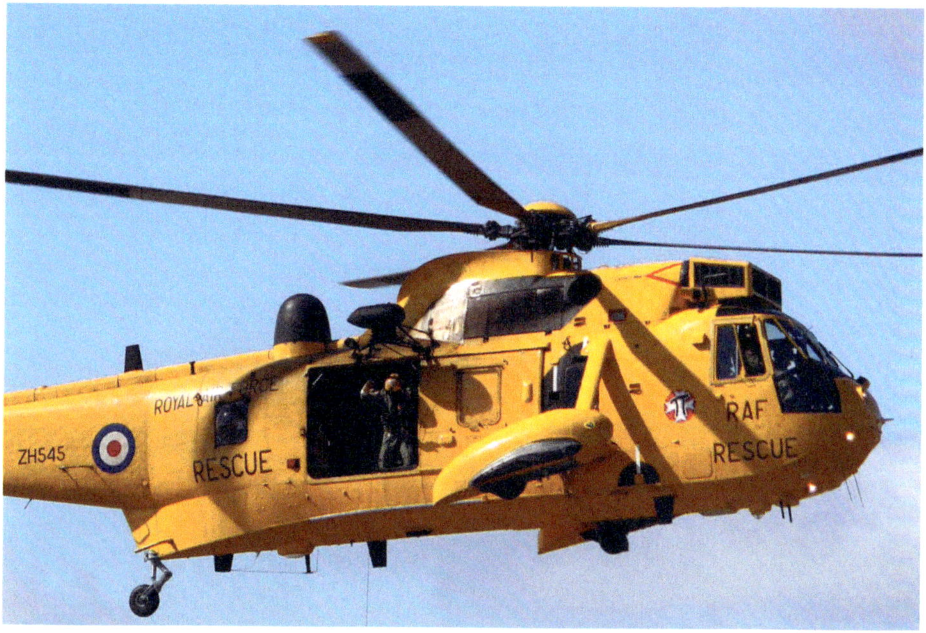

Located on the north Devon coastline at Chivenor, near Barnstaple, until the national demise of the RAF and RN Search & Rescue Sea Kings in late 2015/early 2016 after over forty years of magnificant service, was the RAF's ZH545. It is pictured on exercise over Burnham-on-Sea. 31 August 2014.

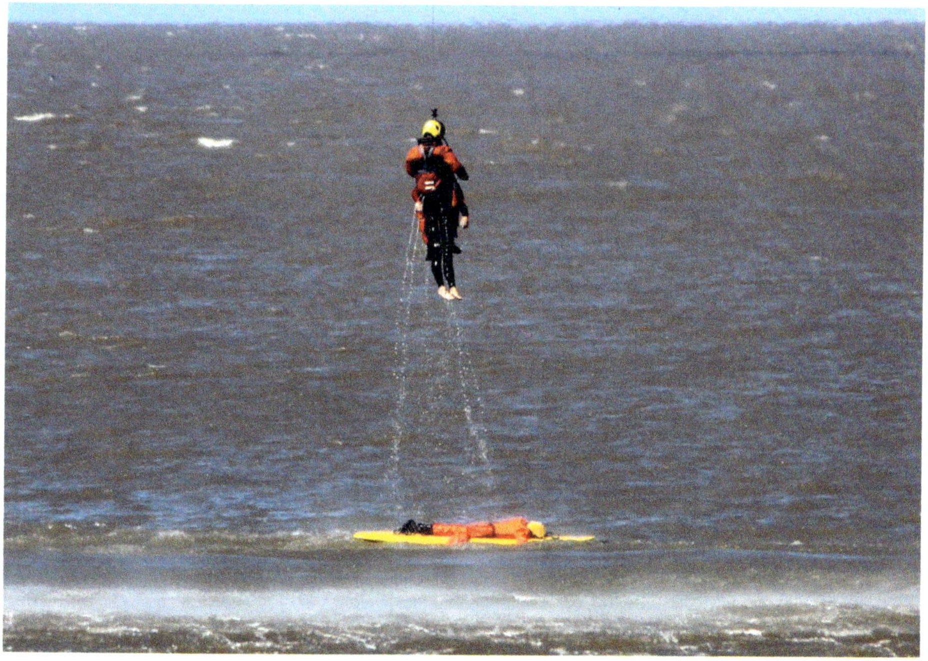

One 'casualty' is plucked out of the water and is being lifted towards the aircraft, a thunderous roar emanating from the Sea King's engines as it maintains its hover position. 31 August 2014.

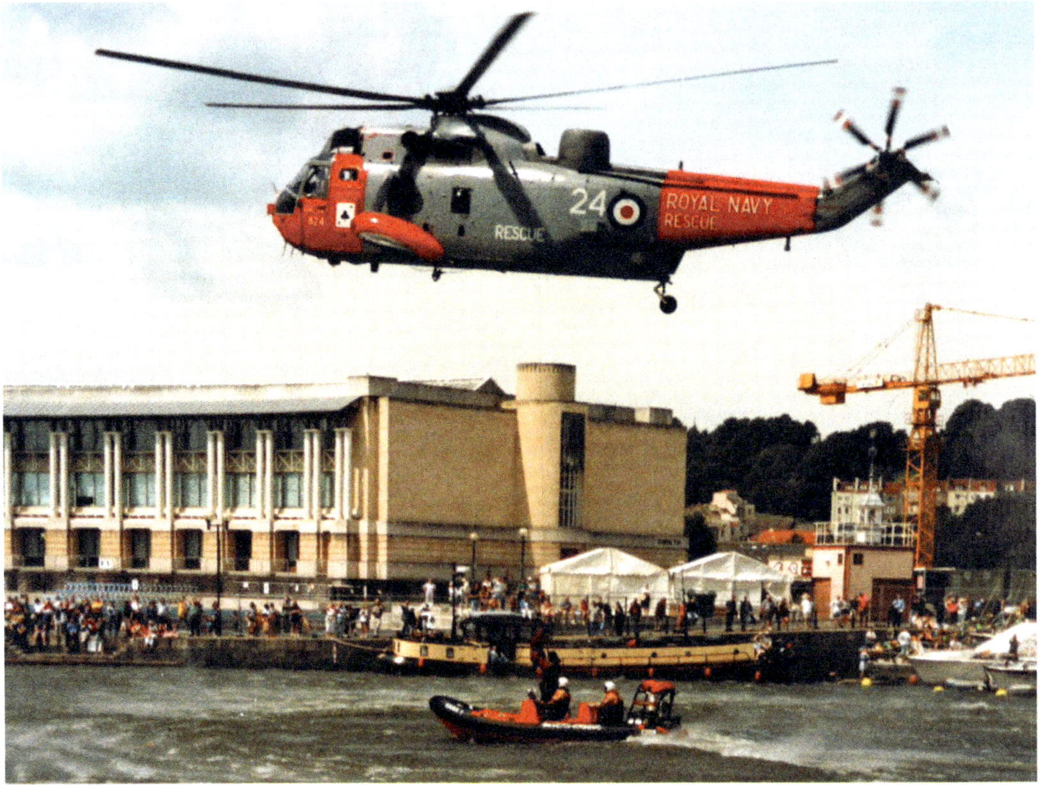

Royal Navy Sea King Search & Rescue helicopter Two-Four from HMS Sea Hawk, the naval land base at Culdrose, near Helston, Cornwall, is pictured in Bristol Harbour with SARA (Severn Area Rescue Association) rigid inflatable boat No. 1, which is carrying out a simulated rescue at the annual harbour festival. HM Coastguard, using Bristow fleet AW189 and Sikorski S-92 aircraft, took over the civilian Search & Rescue role as the military relinquished the task. Bases at Newquay (Cornwall) and St Athan (south Wales) have joined Lee-on-Solent (Hampshire) in providing coverage in the open sea and along the extensive West of England coastline. 25 July 1998.

CHAPTER 3

Fire and Rescue

Never Forgotten

I was both humbled and privileged to have been asked by Fleur's father, Roger, to take the official family photographs at the unveiling of her local memorial on 2 February 1997 in Staple Hill, South Gloucestershire, opposite the site where she lost her life on the morning of Sunday 4 February 1996.

A flashover occurred within a Leo's supermarket, which was deliberately set on fire by a bored security guard on his first day at work there. Fleur, who was posthumously awarded the Queen's Gallantry Medal, died in the intense heat despite the valiant efforts to rescue her by crewmates Rob Seaman, subsequently awarded the George Medal, and Pat Foley, who was awarded the Queen's Commendation for Brave Conduct. Fleur, aged twenty-one and Silver Axe winner on her 1994 recruit's course as top student, was the first female firefighter to die in peacetime in this country.

In a private conversation in 1997 with Roger, requesting his permission to use any images I took of the memorial ceremony, he said: 'Anything that can help draw attention to the need for the fitting of sprinklers to supermarkets will be welcome by me and if publication of any photographs helps then it will be a step I welcome. However, there is one condition to the publishing of any photographs you have taken at today's ceremony. It must not be forgotten that two firefighters from Blaina, Gwent, gave their lives in the line of duty only four days before Fleur gave hers. They must be equally remembered, as must their families.'

That I now do, the opportunity presenting itself in writing this book twenty-two years after promising Roger I would should I ever put anything in print. The house fire in Blaina killed a five-year-old boy who died on the way to hospital. Two retained firefighters, Kevin Lane and Stephen Griffin, both family men, were killed re-entering the blazing building having been wrongly informed a second child was trapped. Tragically, a massive explosion threw them from the upper level to the ground floor.

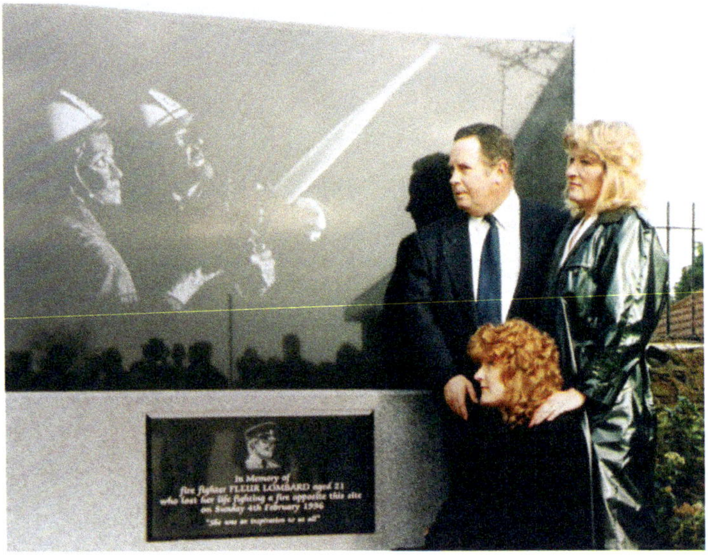
In Memory of
fire fighter FLEUR LOMBARD aged 21
who lost her life fighting a fire opposite this site
on Sunday 4th February 1996

Roger Lombard, his wife Jane and their daughter Rebecca pause for reflection at the unveiling of Fleur's memorial in Staple Hill, South Gloucestershire, opposite the spot where she fell. 2 February 1997.

Aerial Appliances

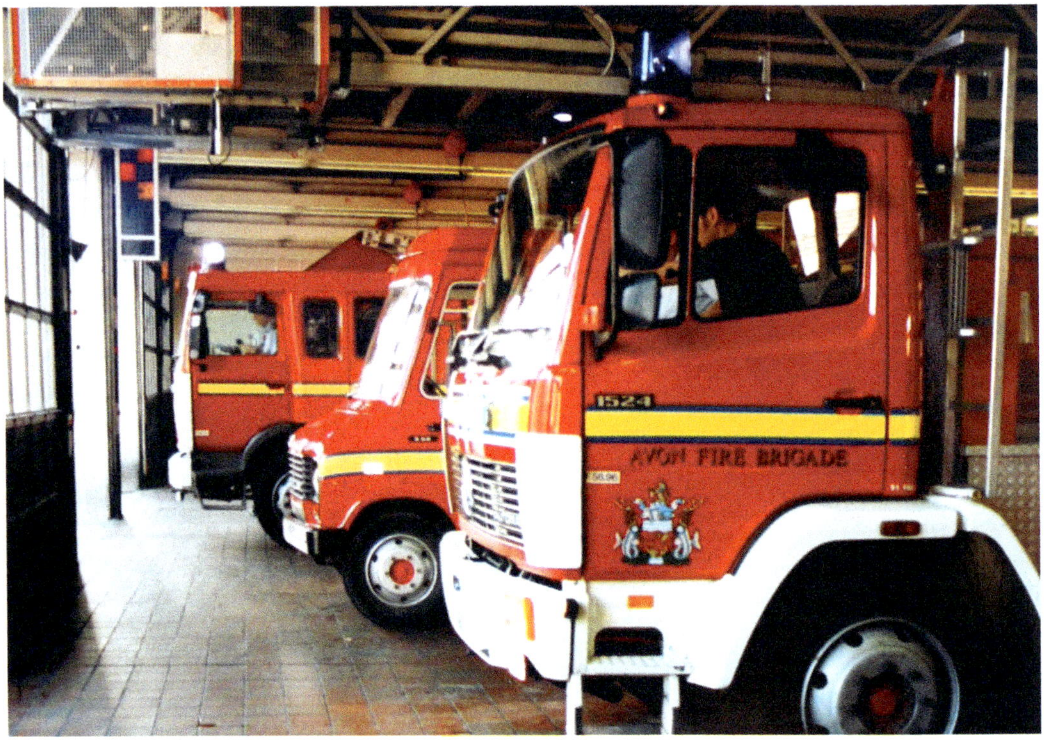
1524
AVON FIRE BRIGADE

Turnout at Bristol's A1 (subsequently renumbered station 09) as a pump departs from a far bay with the turntable ladder N601 LHT (nearest camera) about to follow. At that time the station was running three wholetime pumps, Renault/Saxon Midliners registered M277–279 DOU. 11 November 1997.

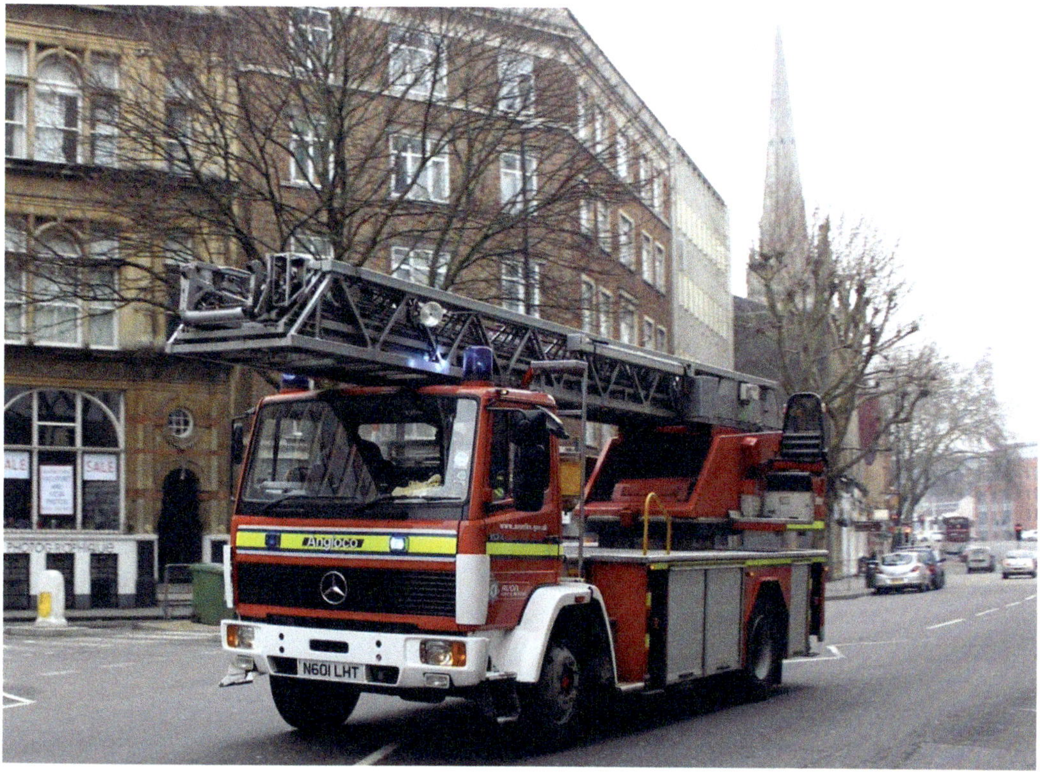

Mercedes/Angloco/Metz turntable ladder N601 LHT charges down Baldwin Street, Bristol, a journey it was to make hundreds of times in the seventeen years it was on the run, all spent at nearby Temple fire station. 2000.

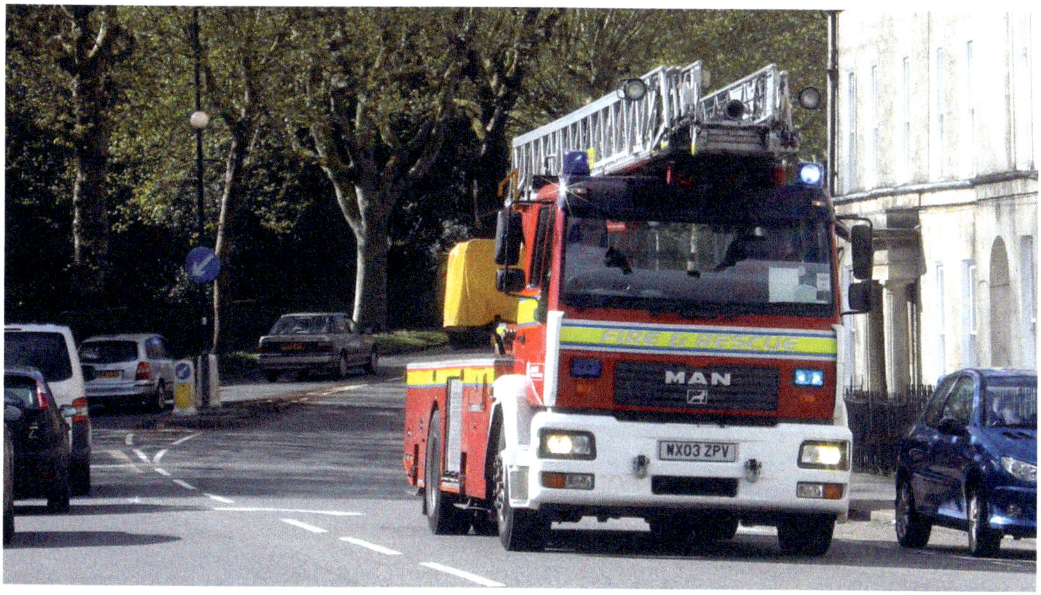

Bath's MAN turntable ladder, WX03 ZPV, gets in its stride, having just turned out from its home station in Bathwick Street. 1 May 2012.

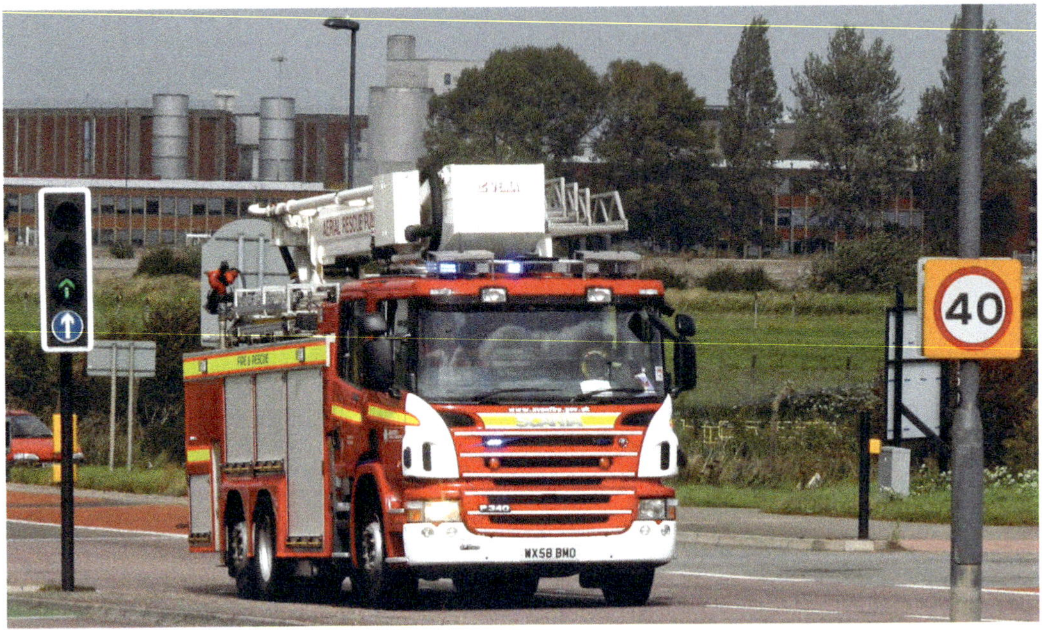

Patchway's Scania/Polybilt/JDC/Vema CARP (Combined Aerial Rescue Pump), WX58 BMO, blasts its way through the traffic lights on the A38 at Filton airfield, inbound towards Bristol. This vehicle was the one used in the original Oxford Die Cast model of a CARP. 2012.

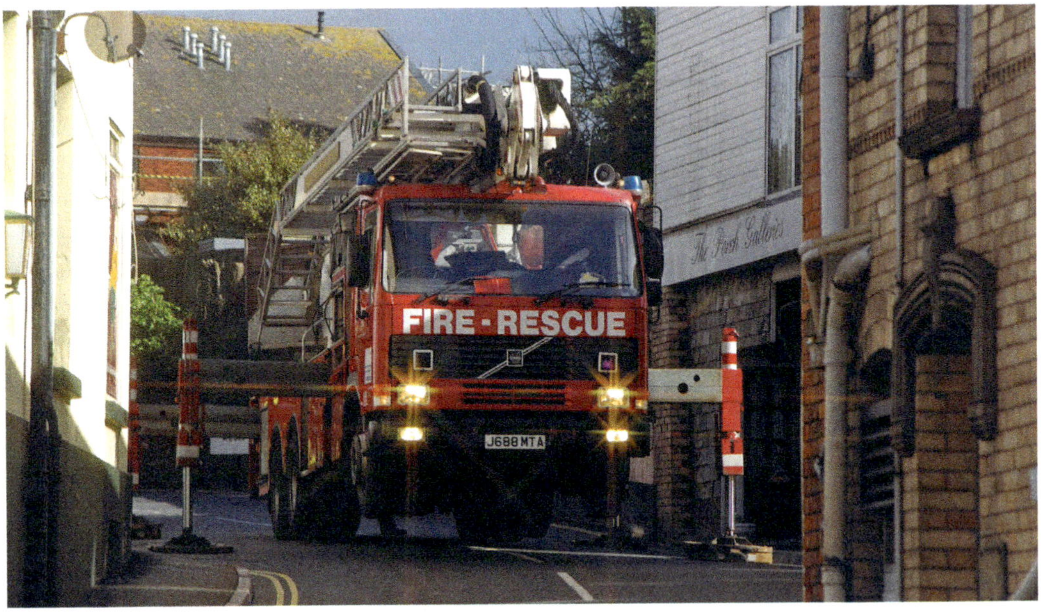

The crew of the Torquay Volvo aerial ladder platform J688 MTA will shortly complete making up their appliance, it having been expertly deployed on the steep, narrow S-bend with adverse camber on the A379 through the town of Dawlish to lower a critically ill patient on a stretcher to ground level. The patient's condition made removal via the building's narrow twisting staircase an impossibility. 3 March 2007.

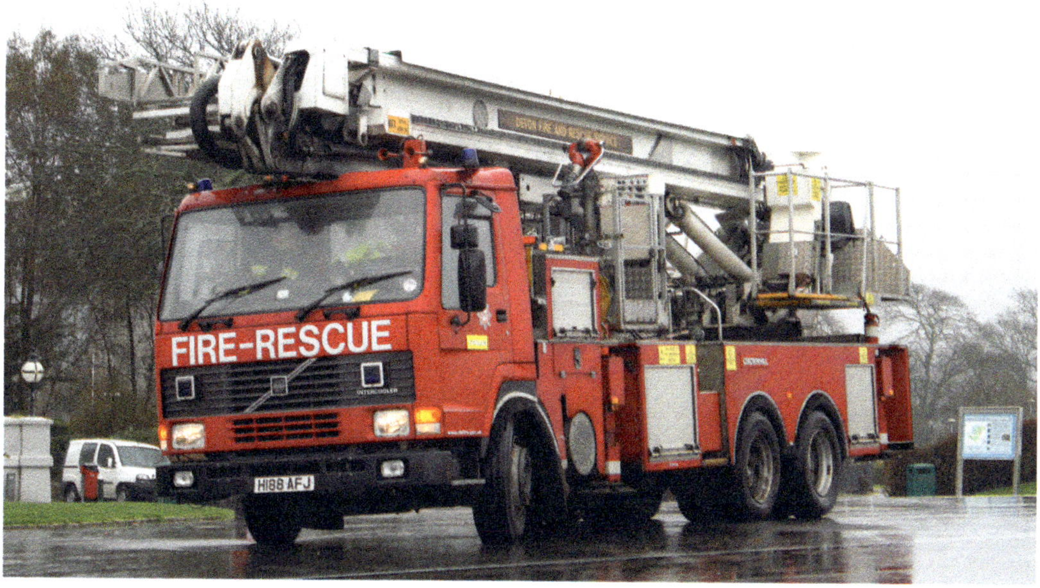

H188 AFJ was used as a photographic platform for official images by the fire and rescue service of a unique handover of six new aerial appliances, one of which would replace this Crownhill-based machine. 22 March 2010.

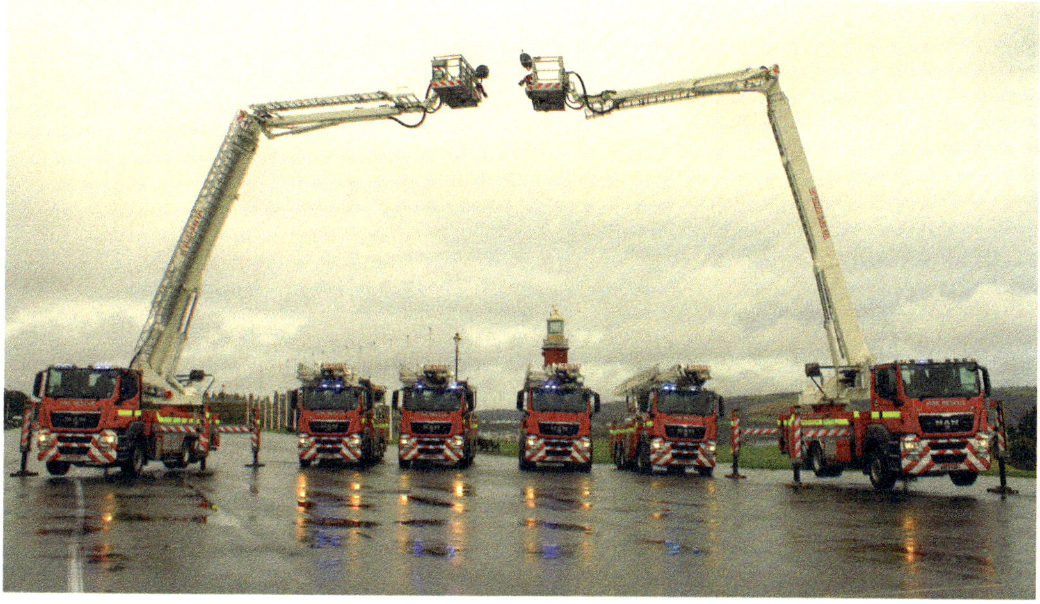

This shot, with Smeaton's Tower in the background on Plymouth Hoe, is never likely to be repeated. It features the official handover in lashing rain and strong wind of six new MAN aerial ladder platform appliances, five destined for Devon & Somerset Fire and Rescue Service, and one for Cornwall FRS. From left to right are WA59 FUF (Crownhill), WA59 FUB (Torquay), WA59 FUG (Exeter), WK59 BPZ (Cornwall), WA59 FUE (Yeovil), and WA59 FUD (Taunton). 22 March 2010.

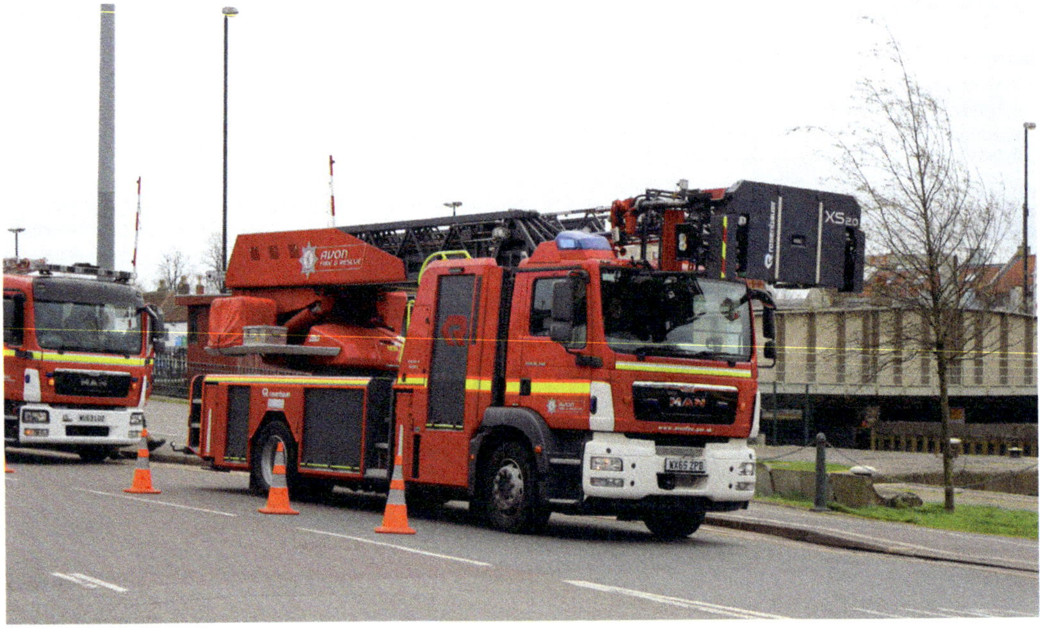

Temple's MAN/Rosenbauer/Metz L32 turntable ladder, WX65 ZPB, pictured with the kind permission of the watch manager at a training session in Bristol's Cumberland Basin. 19 March 2017.

Airport Fire Service

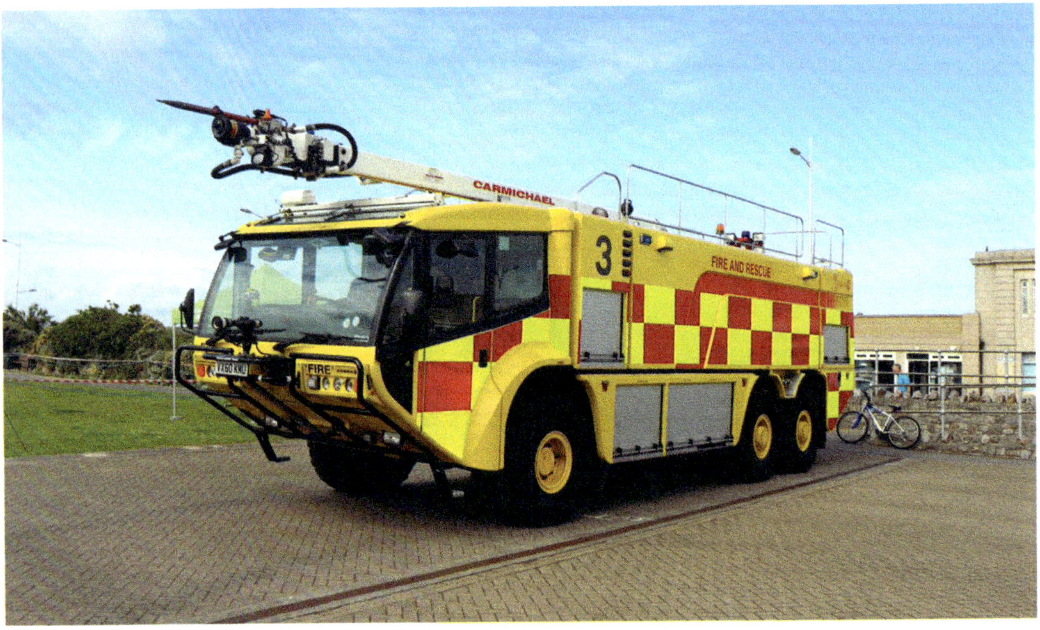

Bristol Airport F&RS brought this mammoth Carmichael Cobra 2 appliance, VX60 KMU, to the Weston-super-Mare 999 day hosted by the town's RNLI. 3 July 2016.

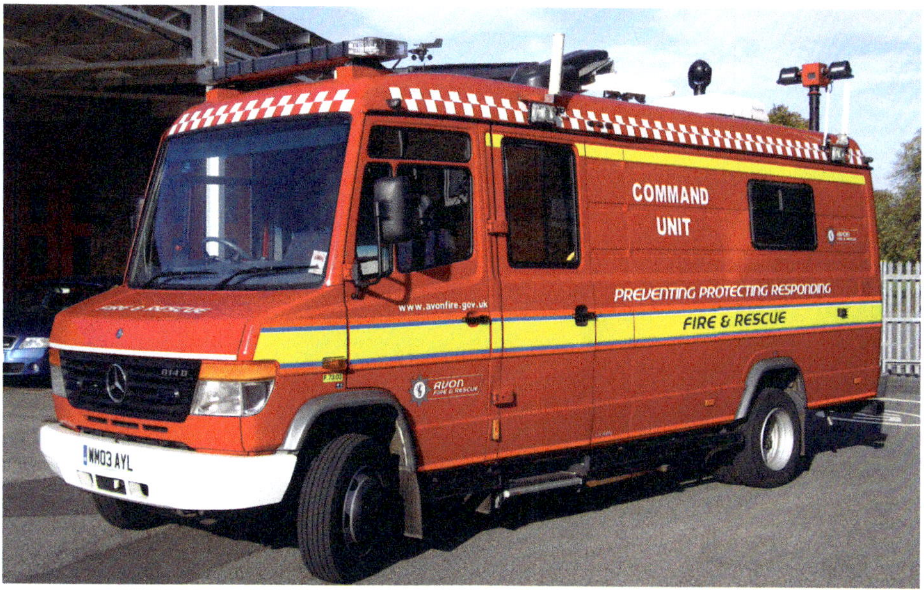

Based at Kingswood fire station, South Gloucestershire, from 2003 until 2018 was Avon's Mercedes 814D/Saxon Command Unit, WM03 AYL. (Image: James Roberts)

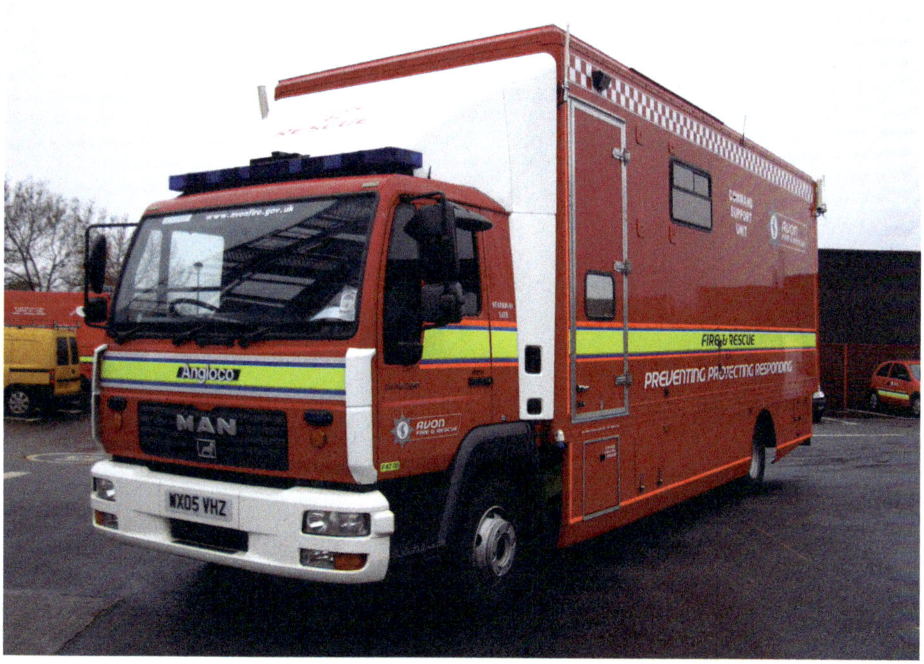

Running in partnership with the Mercedes Command Unit was a 2005 MAN/Angloco Command Support Unit, WX05 VHZ, formerly based at Yate and subsequently at Kingswood. (Image: James Roberts)

Community Fire Education

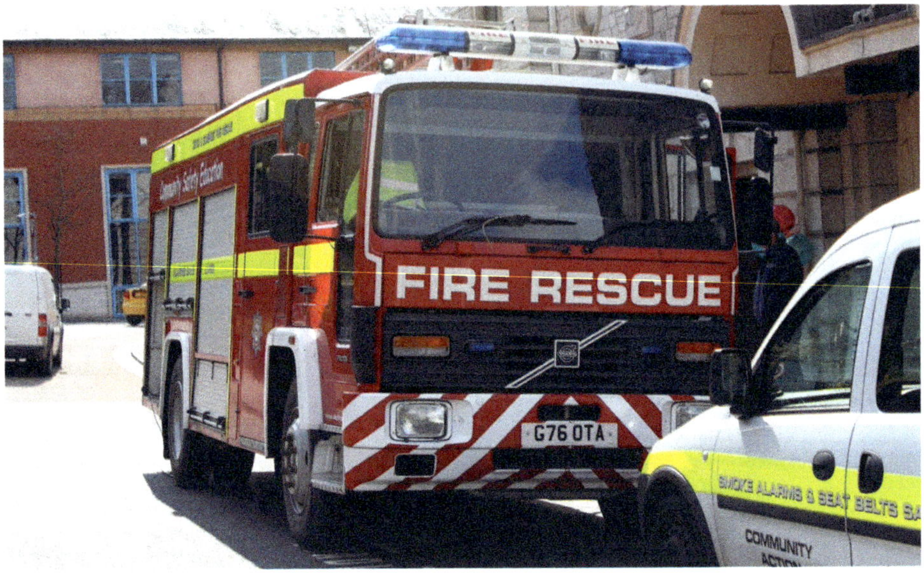

Seen outside Torquay Town Hall, this was one of a batch of seven 1989 Volvo pumps, registered G76–82 OTA, delivered to the Devon brigade. G76 OTA ended its service as a Community Safety Education unit, in which guise it is pictured. The complete rear section was transformed internally into a mini cinema, in which the public could view and receive fire safety advice. 2008.

Co-Responder

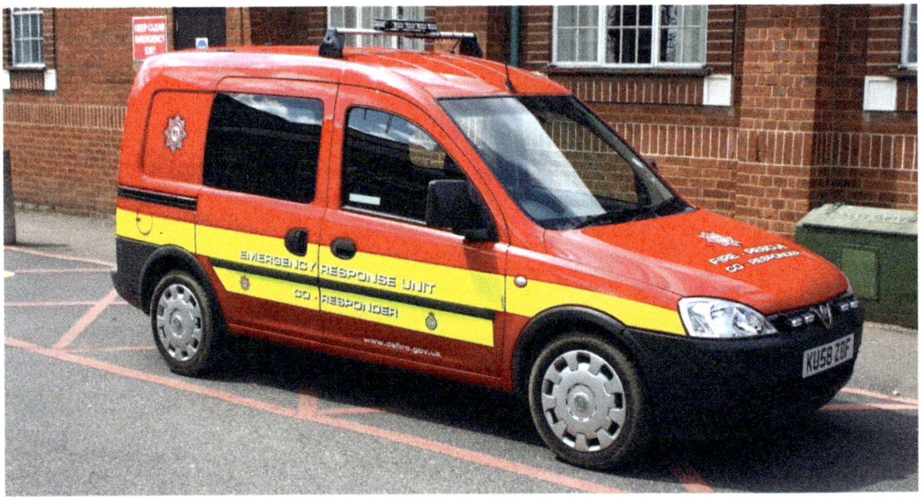

Pictured *c.* 2009 at Topsham fire station was Co-responder Emergency Response Unit KU58 ZBF. Based at twenty fire stations in the county (but not currently at Topsham), these units are an invaluable resource in assisting South Western Ambulance Service by providing initial first aid response, particular in remote rural areas.

Driver Training

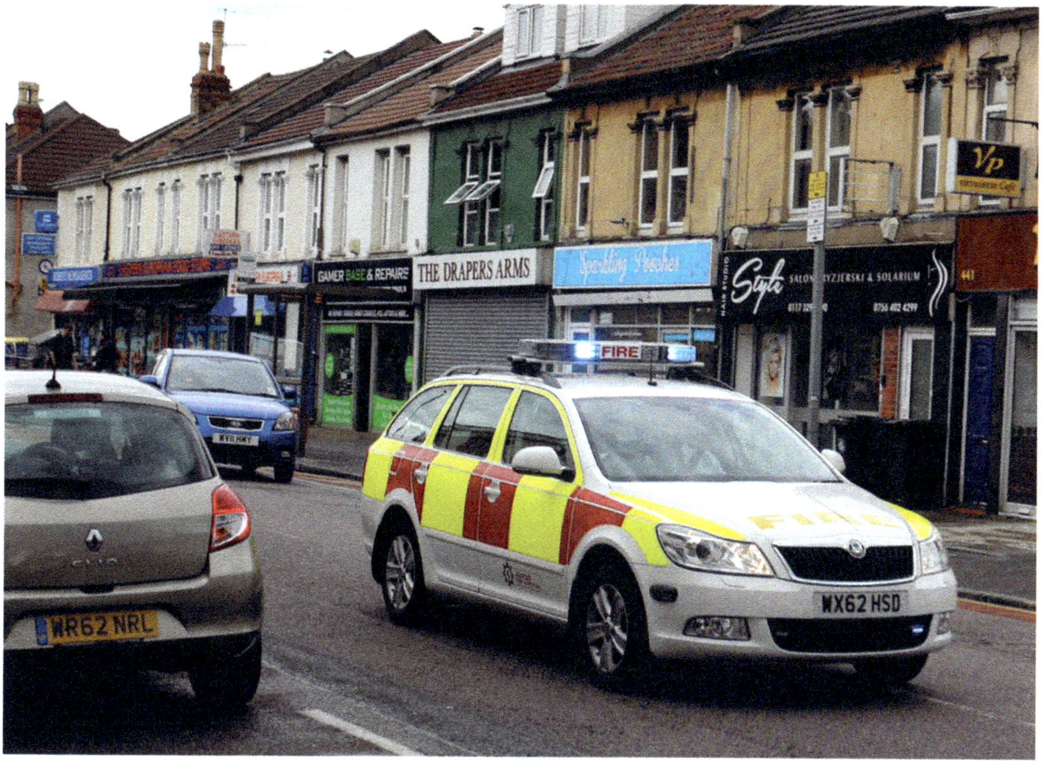

Skoda Octavia 4 x 4 estate WX62 HSD is seen on blue light driver training in Gloucester Road, Horfield, Bristol. 13 July 2016.

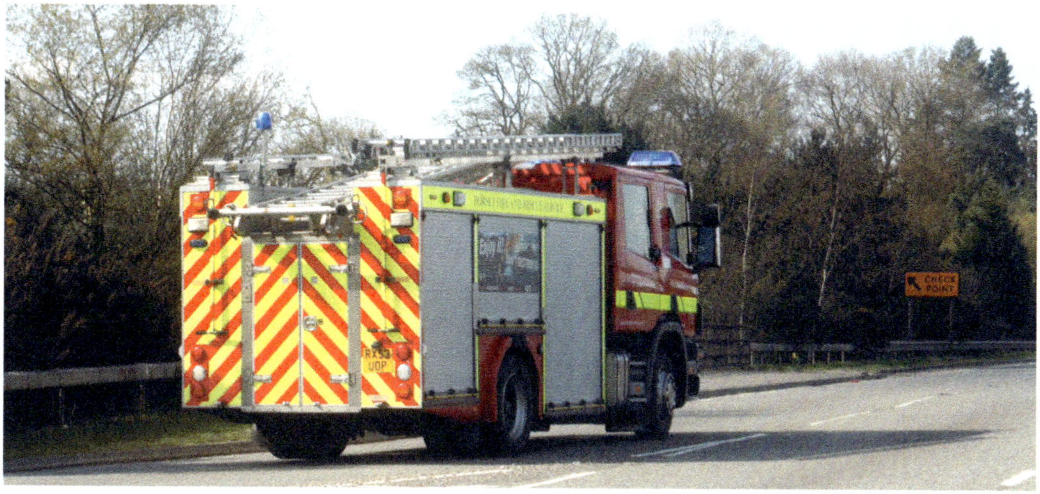

Believed to be on driver training duties, Dorset Scania appliance RX03 UOP is glimpsed near the Hampshire border as it heads westbound in the Ferndown area. The fire and rescue service amalgamated with Wiltshire on 1 April 2016. This image is from 2011. (Image: Margaret Boulter)

Fuel Bowser

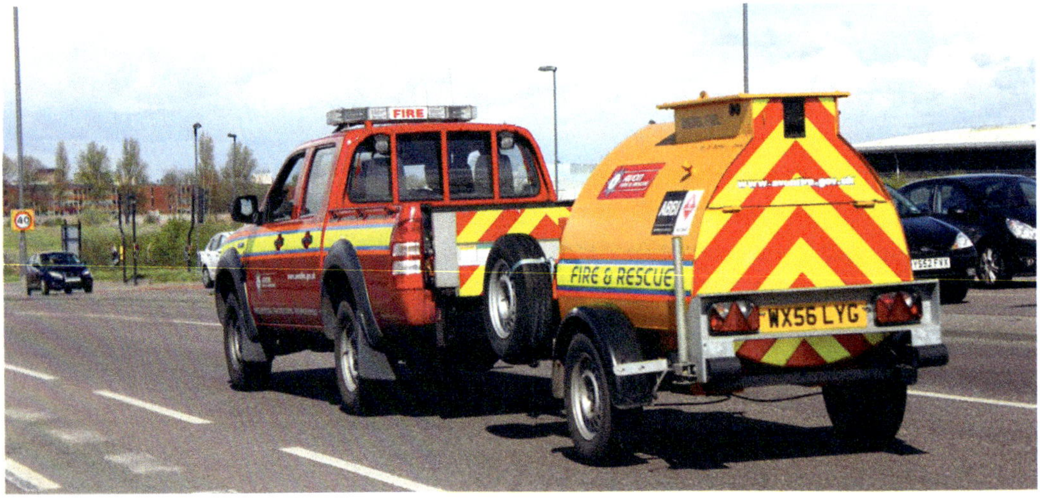

Protracted incidents with appliances working continuously may require additional fuel. Resources exist at strategic locations throughout Avon FRS to allow fuel to be transported as needed. Workshop's Ford Ranger WX56 LYG heads towards Patchway, towing one of ten bowsers in the brigade. 2013.

Hose Layer

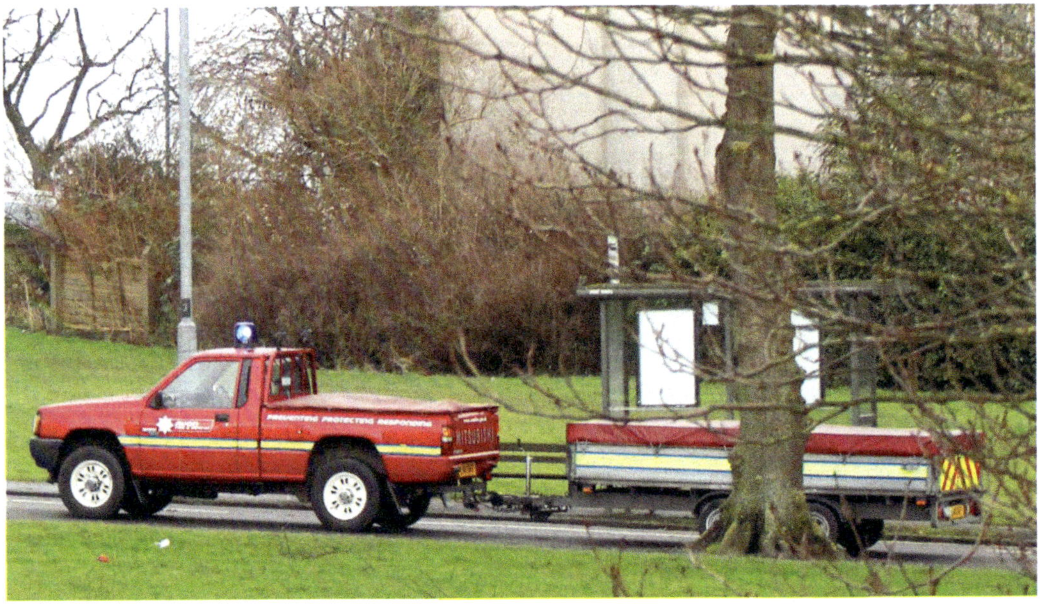

Southmead fire station, Bristol, was home throughout the vehicle's life to 1993 registered Mitsubishi L200 4 x4 L411 SHT and its hose layer trailer. Covering just 18,600 miles by 2015 it retained its original two-tone air horn, giving it a very distinctive sound when mobilised on the blue light. It is pictured on one of its rare shouts as it climbs Wellington Hill West, Horfield. 10 January 2015.

Pumping Appliances

With slight variations in the equipment they carry, appliances are known as pumps or water tenders, with the word 'ladder', when added, generally indicating a 13.5-metre ladder is carried. Wheeled escape ladders were phased out nationally in the late 1980s/early 1990s.

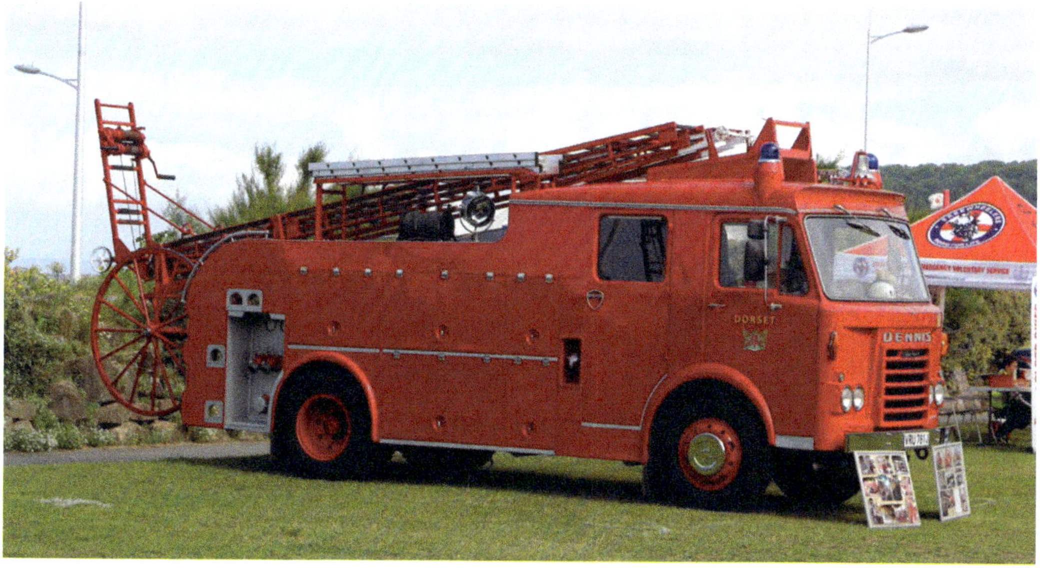

The sound of the clanging bell, the noise of the vehicle's engine under acceleration and the rattling of the escape ladder in its mountings was indeed one the older generation will readily recall! Former Dorset (Bournemouth) Dennis F108 pump escape VRU 781J, in immaculate condition, is pictured at Weston-super-Mare. 3 July 2016.

Weston-super-Mare fire station used to house a Dennis pump escape but not this superbly preserved 1983/84-registered Dennis machine, A253 HPE with a 50-foot wheeled escape, which is seen driving along Beach Road in the town. It belonged in service with Hertfordshire County Council Fire Brigade. 3 July 2016.

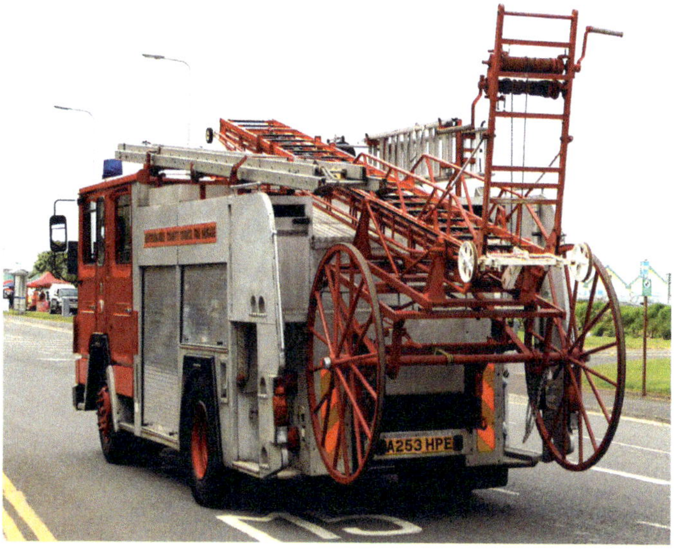

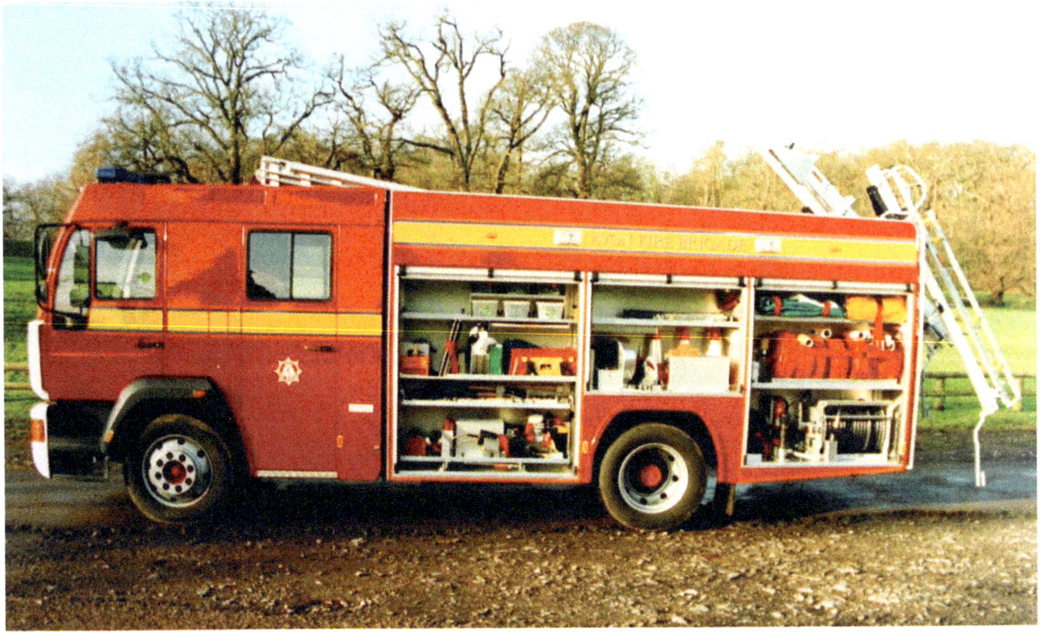

This is R648 BHU, the first MAN/Saxon pump in the Avon brigade. Seen at Ashton Court estate soon after delivery, it was stationed at Radstock, where it spent its entire service with Avon. It ran as a water tender ladder (WrL) fitted with a 13.5-metre three-piece main ladder rather than as a water tender (WrT), the latter designation which would have seen it run with a 10.5-metre two-piece main ladder in Avon. 14 September 1998.

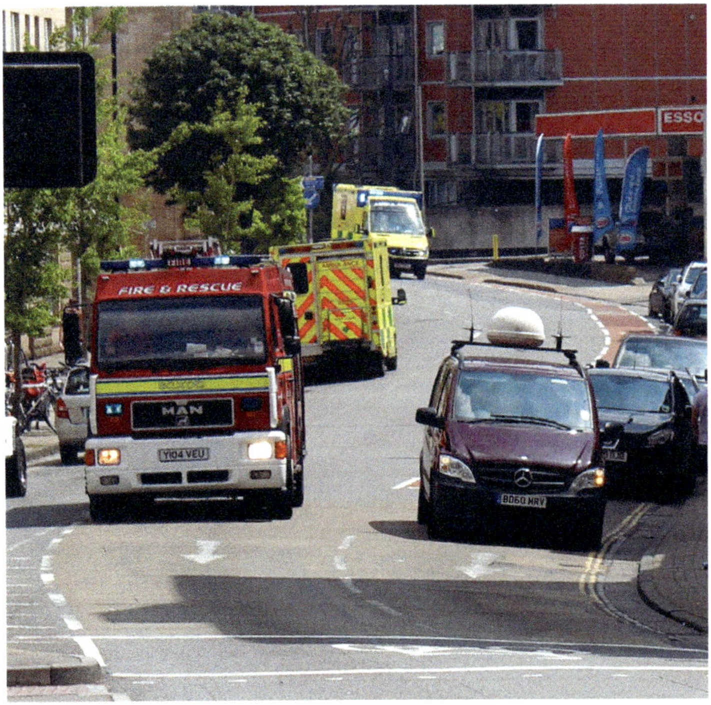

A reserve appliance that stood in for Temple's WrL, Y104 VEU gathers speed as it blasts through Park Row, soon to be followed by an ambulance attending the same emergency. Travelling in the opposite direction, another ambulance heads for the nearby Bristol Royal Infirmary. 1 June 2014.

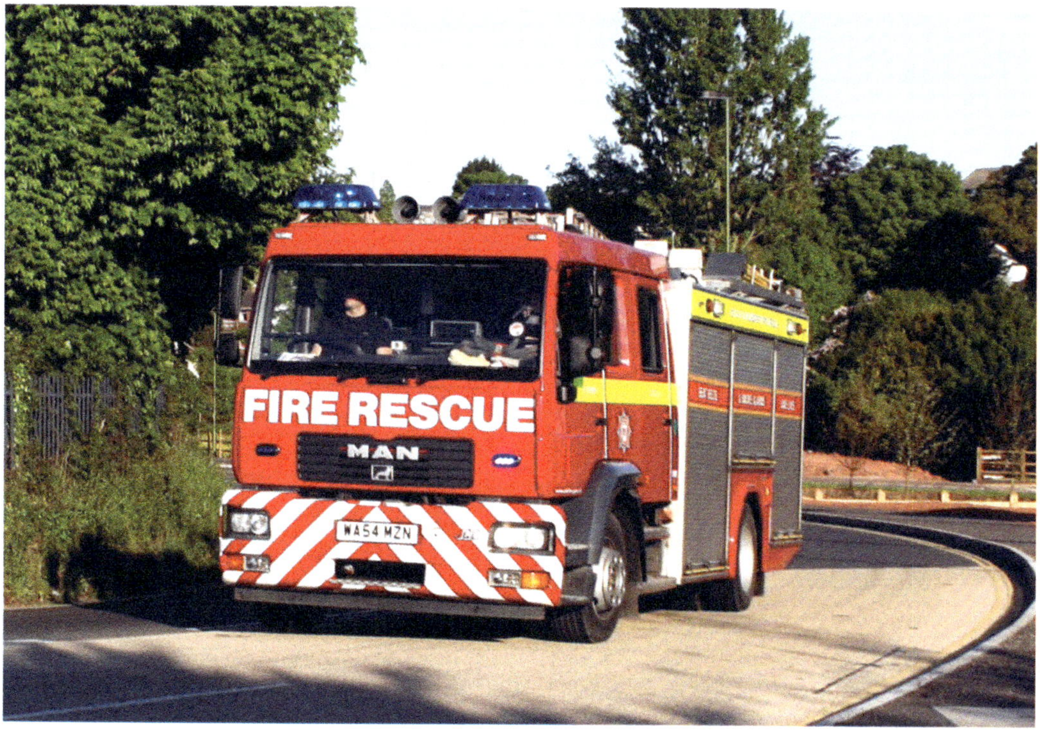

A Torquay appliance on a shout backing up a neighbouring station, WA54 MZN is about to join the A380 Torquay Road to head towards Newton Abbot. 2009.

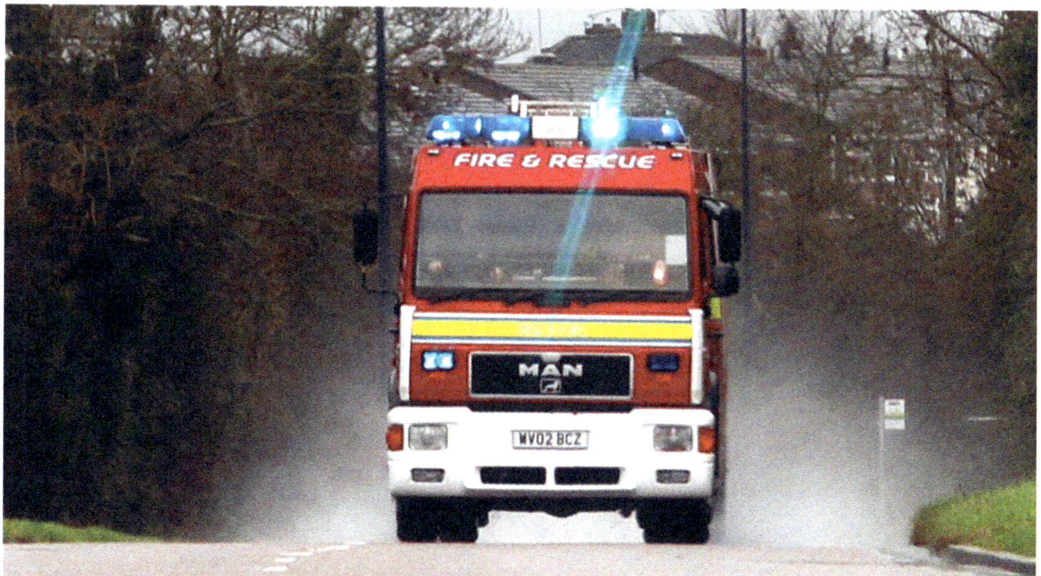

A reserve appliance on the run that damp day from Patchway fire station, South Gloucestershire, was WV02 BCZ storming up Highwood Road, spray flying as the appliance gathers speed. 10 January 2016. (Image: Margaret Boulter)

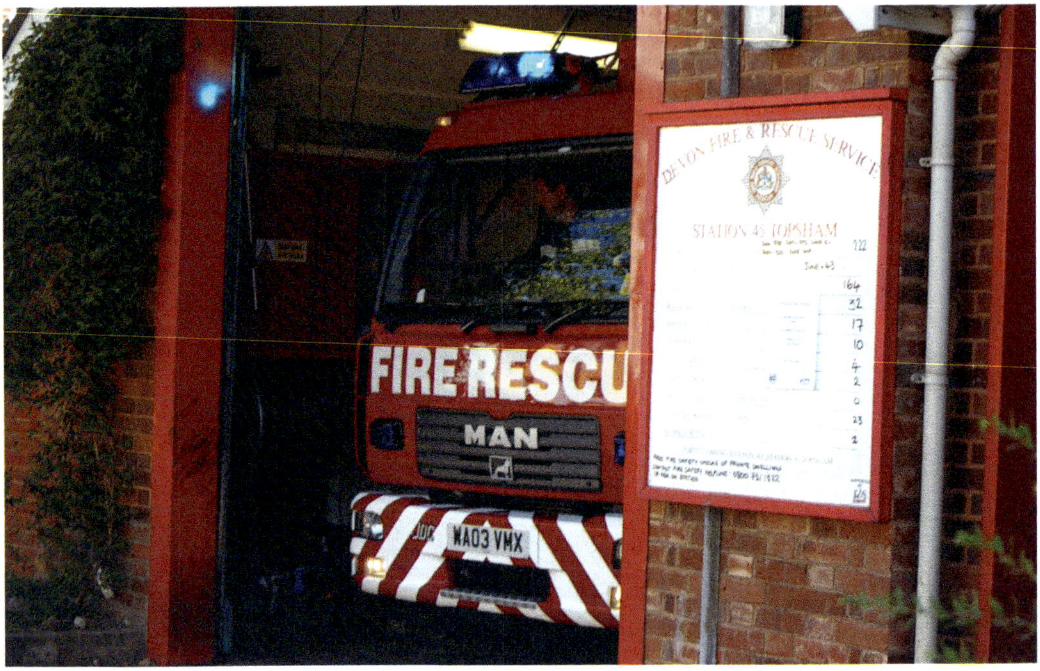

WA03 VMX, the second of two pumps about to turn out on a shout from the Topsham retained fire station located on the south eastern outskirts of Exeter. An excellent innovation on the outer wall between the bays is a public information board showing the number and type of incidents attended during the year. July 2006.

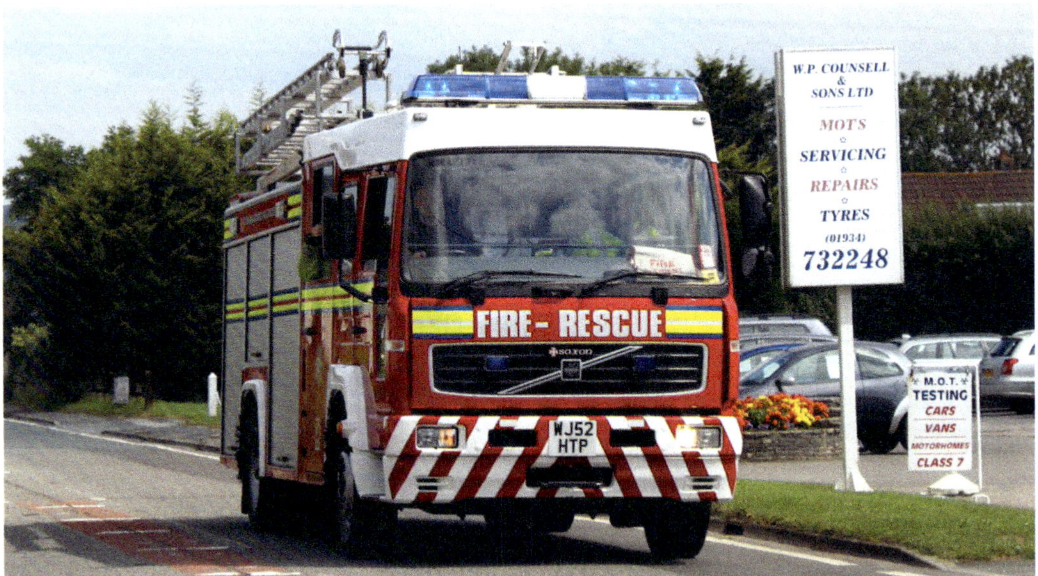

Cheddar's Volvo/Saxon water tender ladder is making good progress on a long straight section of the A38 through Lower Weare, Somerset, as it responds to an emergency. 17 August 2015. (Image: Margaret Boulter)

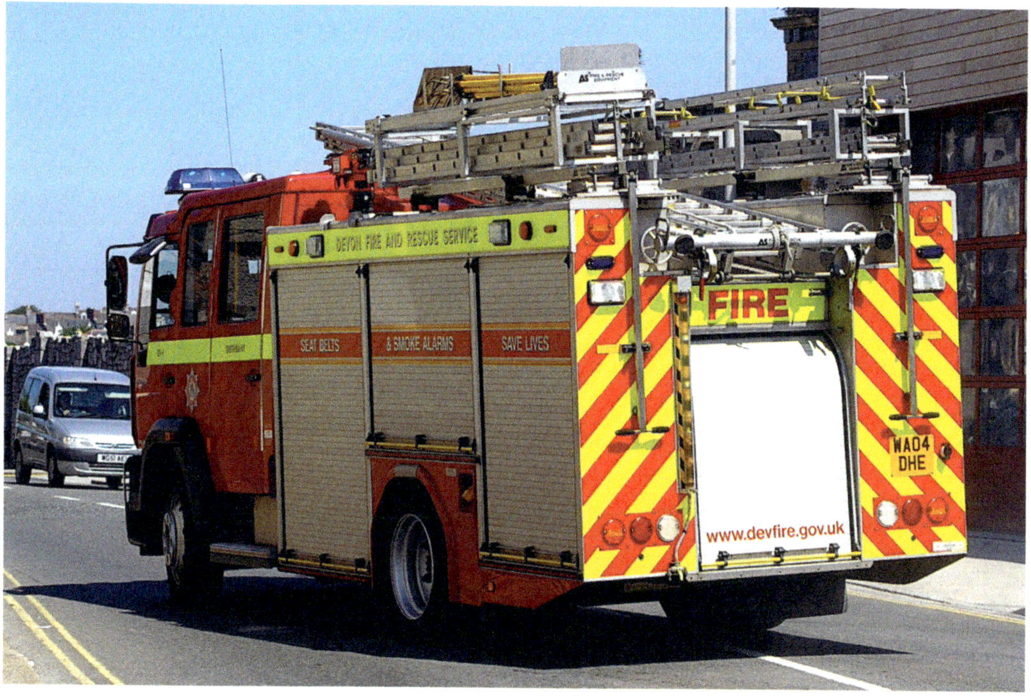

A gleaming Greenbank-based MAN WrL leaves its newly rebuilt home station to go mobile on routine tasks in central Plymouth. 15 July 2006.

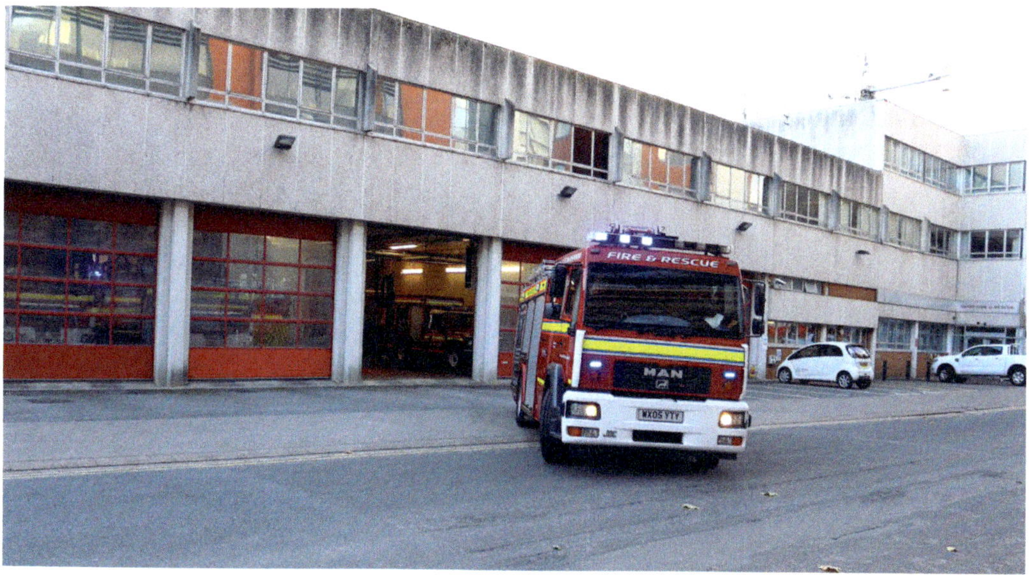

Temple was a nine-bay station when opened in 1973 and was later reduced to seven bays to create aditional office space. Reserve appliance WX05 YTY (ex-Speedwell and ex-Thornbury) performed one of the final turnouts from the forty-three-year old station, the new five-bay central Bristol station opening on the morning of 7 November 2016 two days after this image was taken.

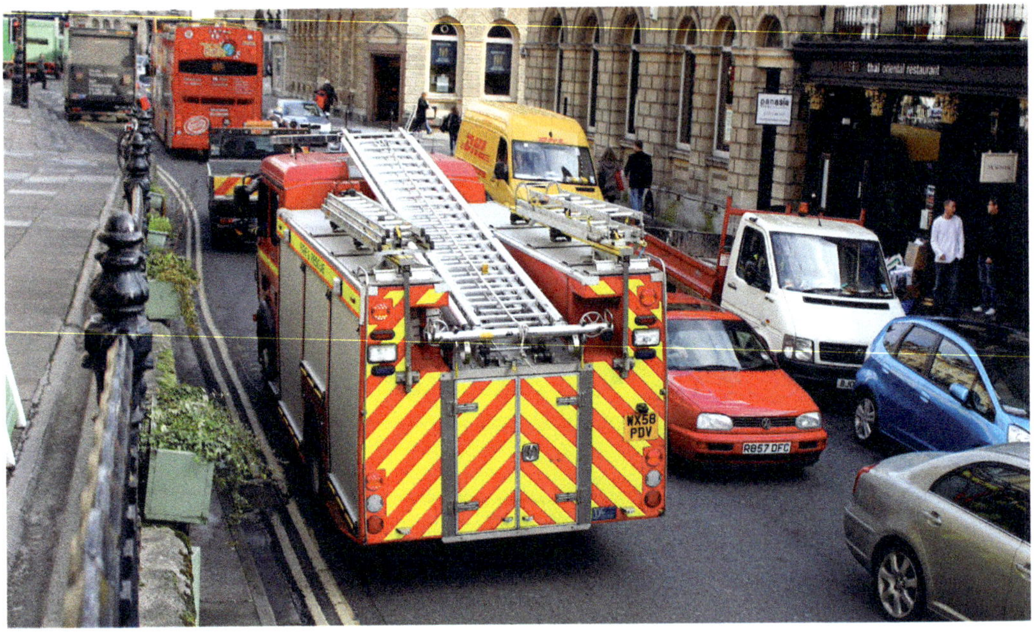

Following a Bath Bus Company tour bus (who operate delightful and interesting open top routes through the famous city) WX58 PDV, the Bath retained crew WrL, is seen heading along George Street at normal road speed. 2012.

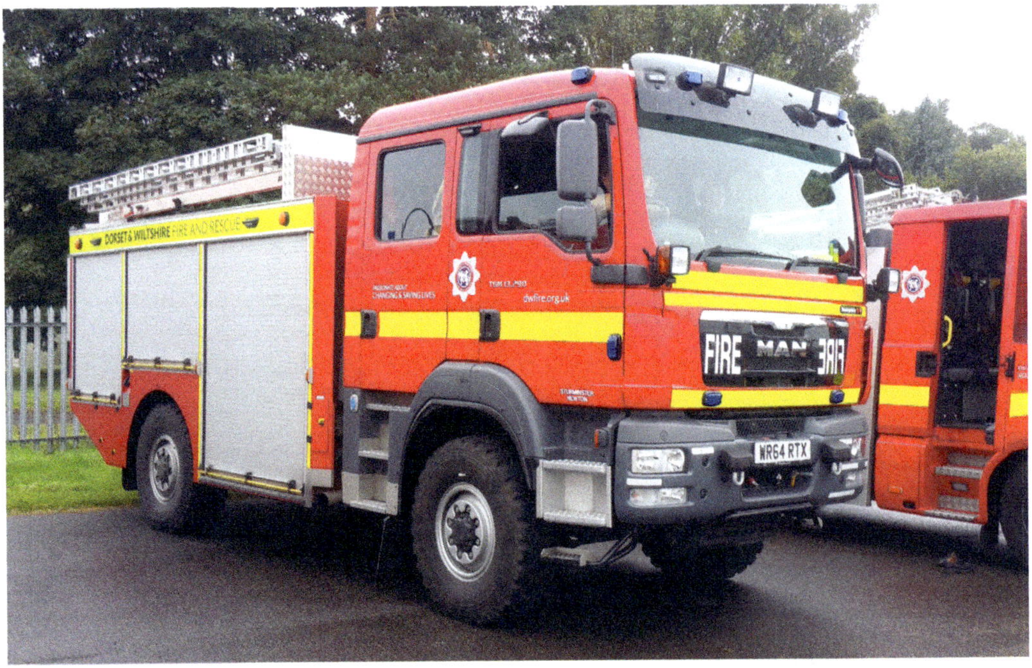

Dorset & Wiltshire FRS 4 x 4 MAN/Emergency One off-road pump WR64 RTX, stationed at Sturminster Newton, near Blandford Forum in Dorset, was one of the exhibits at the September 2017 and 2018 Kemble 999 Show. (Image: Matt Holmes)

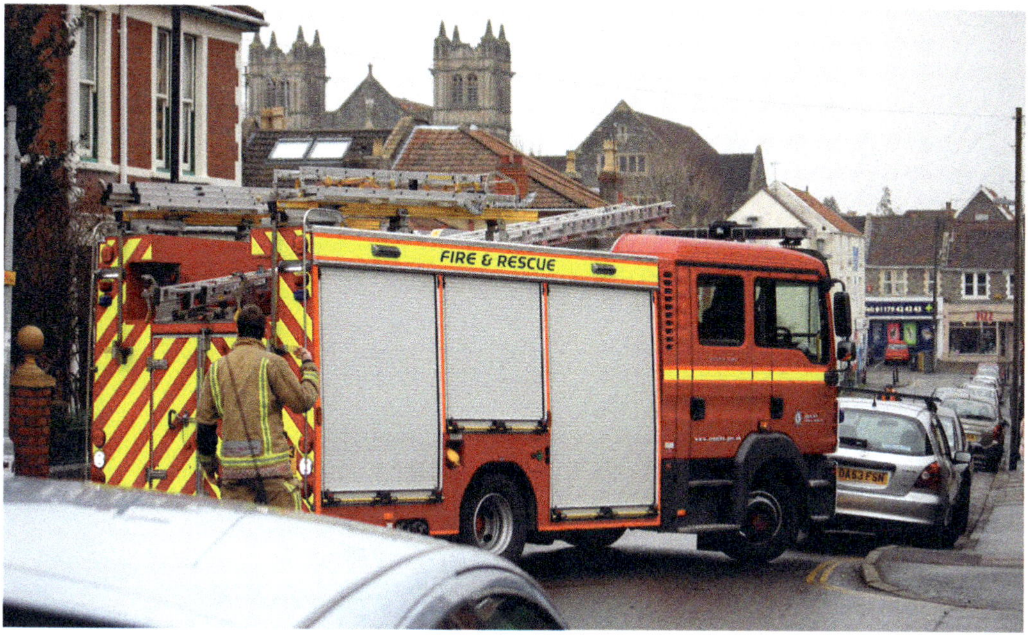

Fortunately this MAN/Polybilt/JDC water tender, WU63 LUZ, was trying to return to its home station at Temple after a fire call to Bristol Prison rather than mobilising to another incident. Due to parked vehicles, trying to turn onto Bishop Road in a free-flowing movement proved impossible. 13 March 2015.

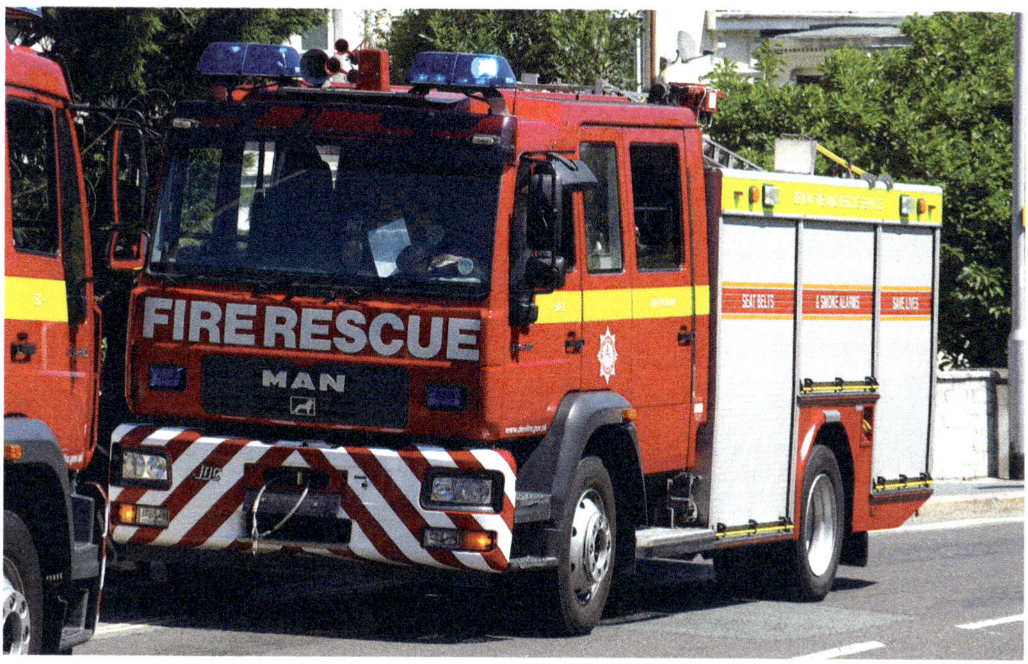

Greenbank's water tender, WA53 PUK, at a small animal rescue in Alexandra Road, Mannamead, Plymouth. 15 July 2006.

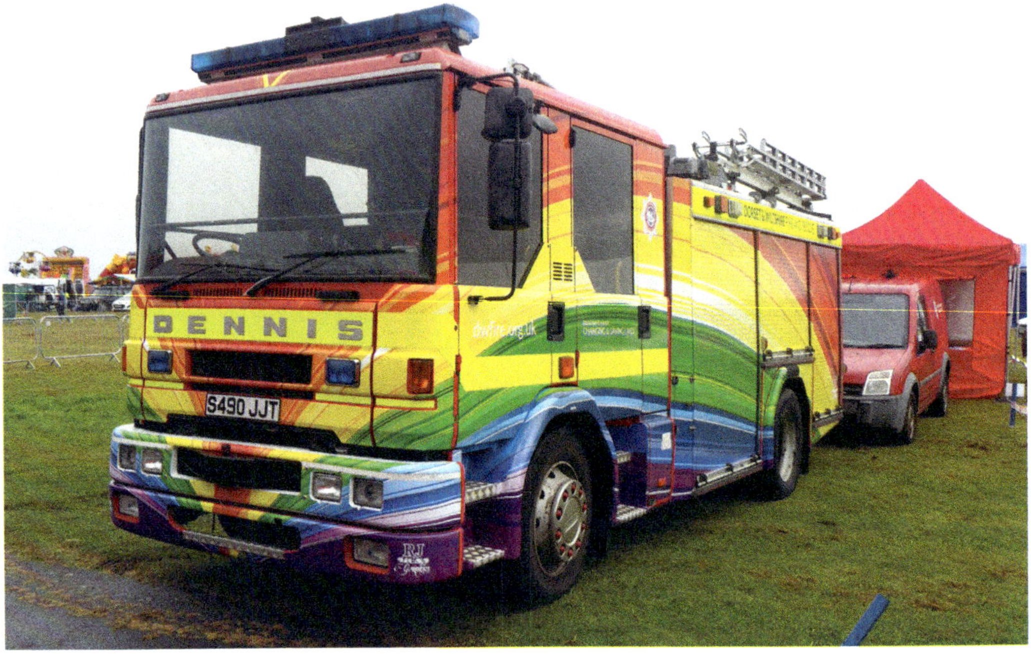

Dorset & Wiltshire FRS Dennis Sabre S490 JJT is seen in the now familiar rainbow colours portraying diversity, equality and inclusion for all. September 2017. (Image: Matt Holmes)

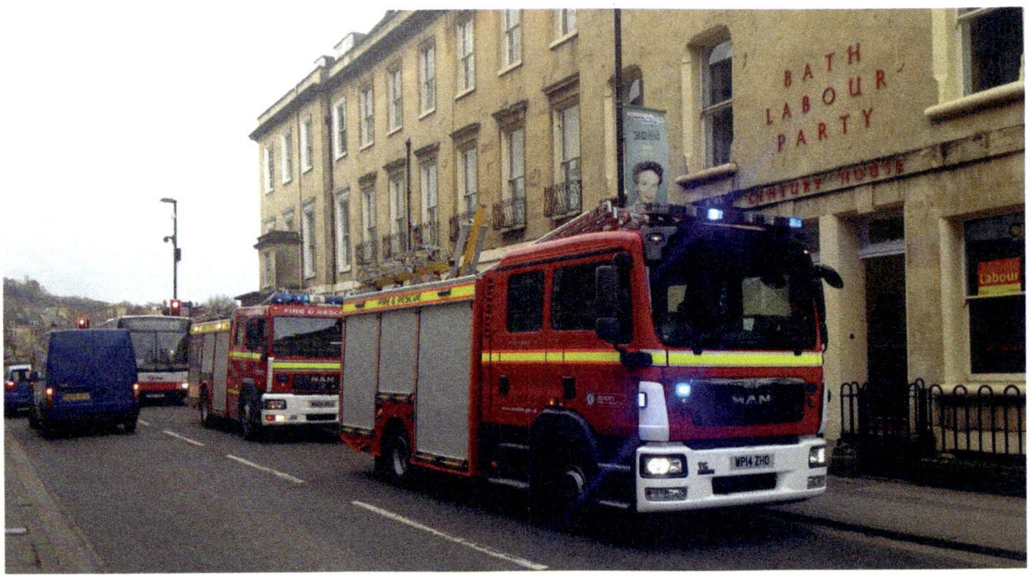

Despite being parked outside a central Bath address, both appliances were stationed elsewhere. WP14 ZHO is the WrL from the wholetime crewed station at Brislington and WU04 HYJ was the retained crewed WrL from Keynsham. Both stations amalgamated on 19 April 2016 to become a new wholetime station at Hicks Gate, halfway between Bristol and Bath. 24 February 2015. (Image: Martin S. Curtis)

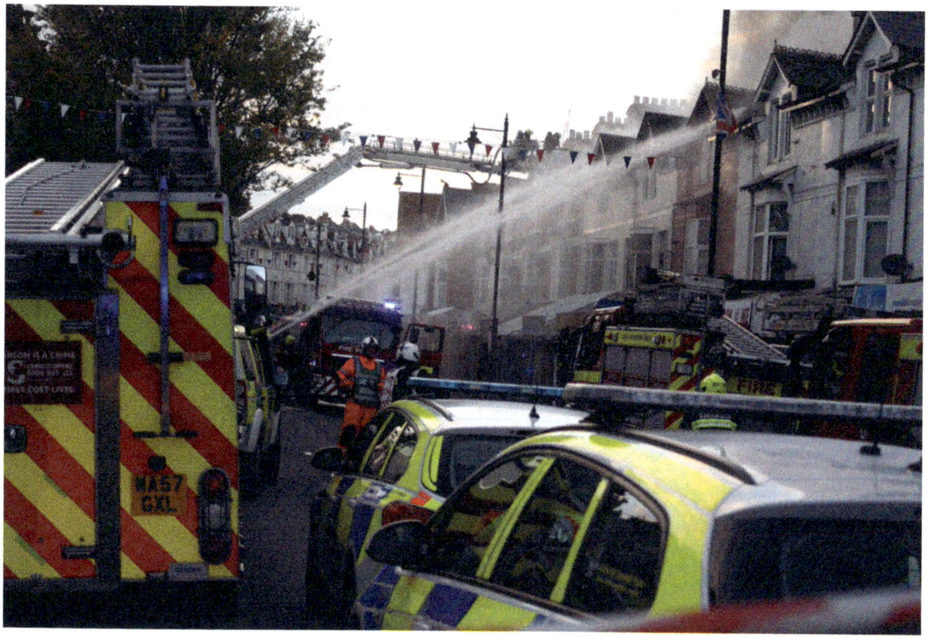

The late afternoon saw fire break out in the ducting of a fish and chip shop extraction system in Torbay Road in the heart of Paignton. This rapidly spread via the roof void to a total of five properties. Jets are in action from Torquay's aerial appliance and several of the sixteen pumping appliances in attendance. 11 October 2018. (Image: Matt Holmes)

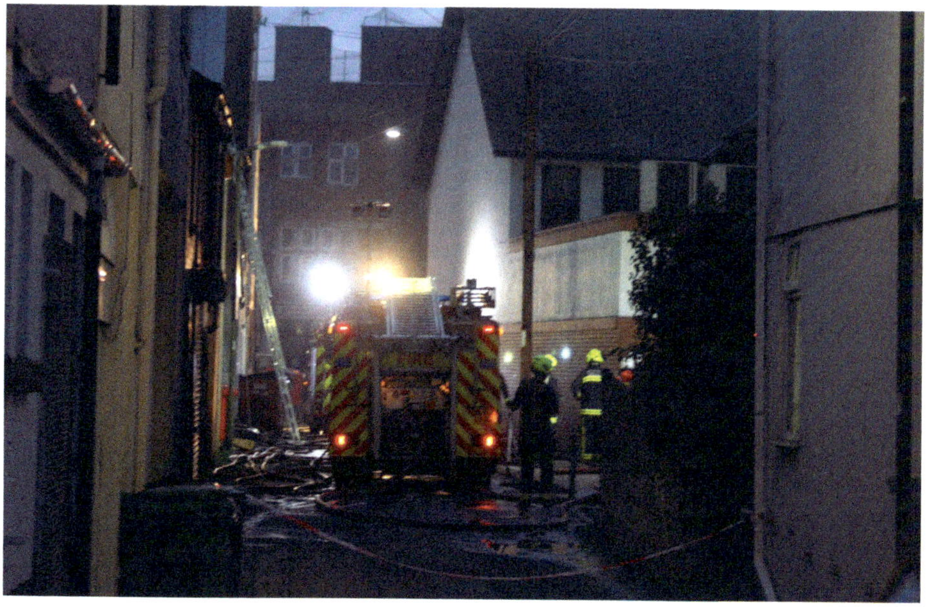

Many of the crews of supporting pumps were required for breathing apparatus purposes. However, in this image taken in Parkside Road at the side of the affected buildings, two pumps are surrounded by a mass of hose lines silhoutted in the temporary lighting from the leading appliance. 11 October 2018. (Image: Matt Holmes)

Rescue Pump

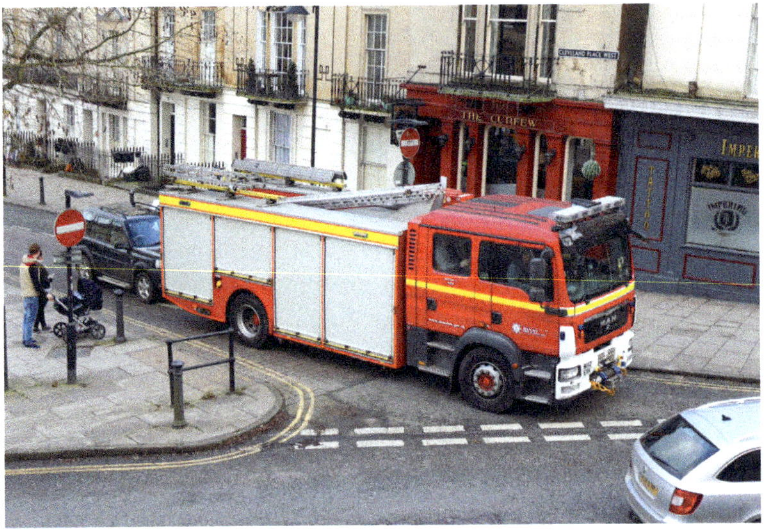

Bath's Rescue Pump (RP), WU12 EXK, fitted with 13.5-metre ladder, pauses at Cleveland Place to join the A4 London Road. Unlike the majority of the pumps within the brigade, Avon's four MAN RPs (based at Avonmouth, Bath, Temple and Weston-super-Mare) are fitted with an additional side locker and front-mounted winch. 21 January 2016.

Rescue Tenders

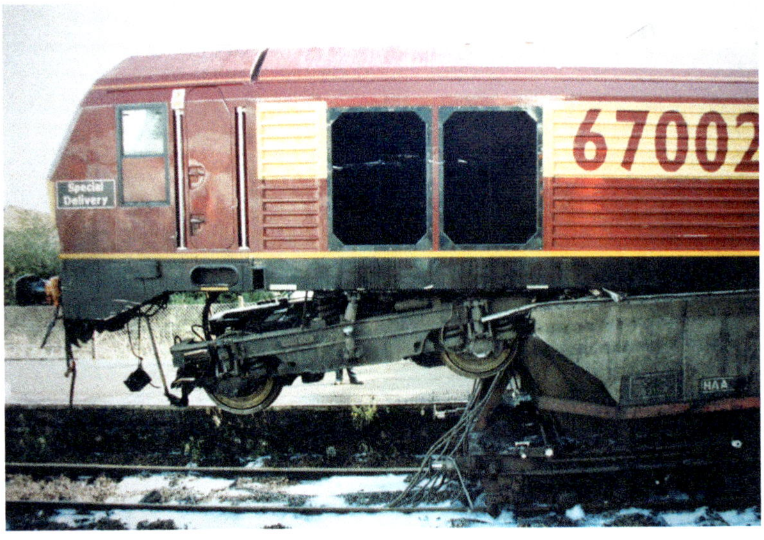

At 03.41 hours, No. 67002 *Special Delivery,* the locomotive of a night mail train, literally took off at 50 mph as it ploughed into the back of a slow-moving coal train. Foam blankets were laid as a precautionary measure, the locomotive's fuel tank capable of holding 5,400 litres of diesel. Four pumps, a rescue tender and an operational support unit with additional foam supplies were in attendance. 1 November 2000.

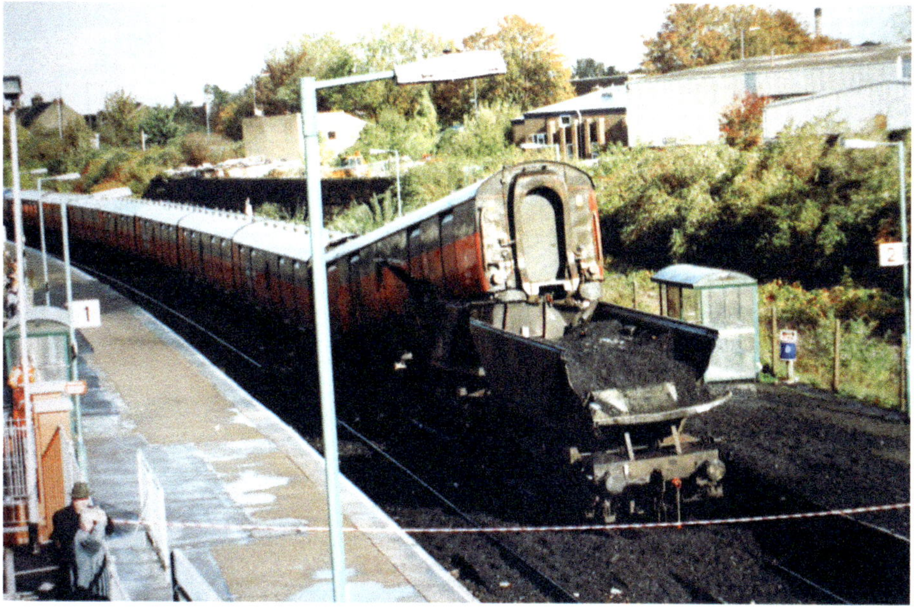

In the collision the locomotive broke from its mail coaches, rearing up in the air and, unbelievedly, landing on top of moving coal wagons which came to a sudden halt 100 metres later when the wagons and their uninvited 90-ton 'guest' struck the A420 road bridge at Lawrence Hill railway station, Bristol. A small fire in the locomotive was quickly extinquished and, somewhat miraculously, the driver only suffered comparitively minor injuries.

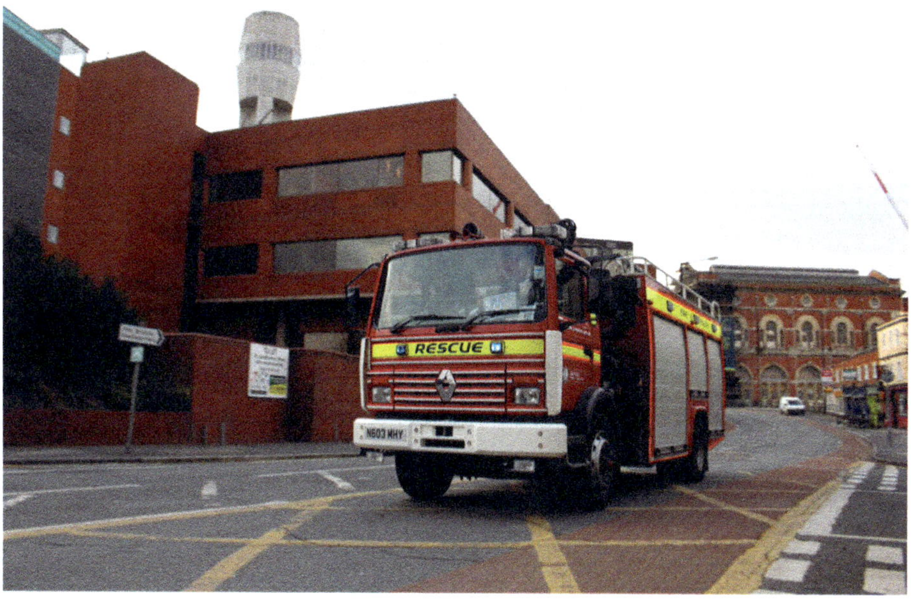

On the initial attendance to the rail crash fourteen years earlier was Temple's 1996 Renault/Saxon rescue tender, N603 MHY, fitted with a crane behind the cab. It served all of its working life at Temple before disposal to the Gambia F&RS. February 2014.

Road/Rail Rescue Unit

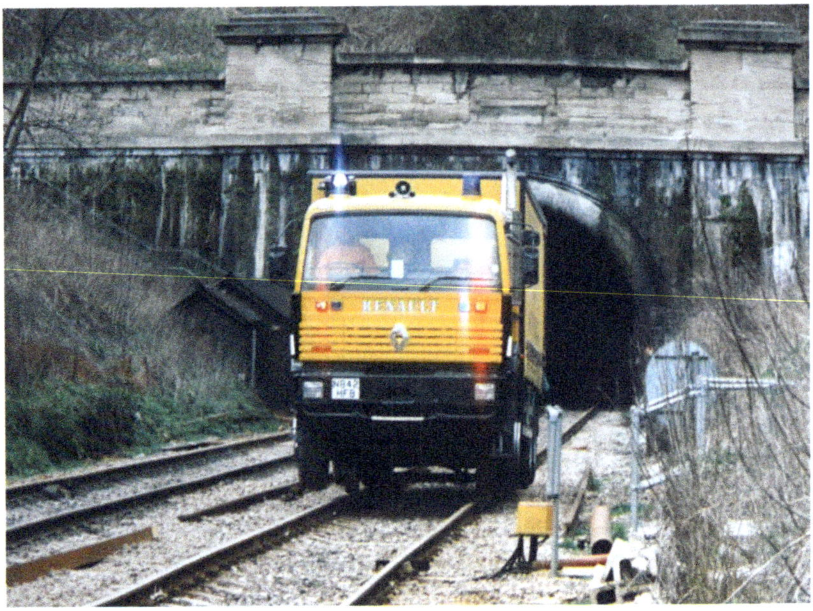

As an invited photographer at the exercise, the author was able to capture the Renault Maxter G300-26D road/rail rescue unit N842 HFB as it emerged on the blues from the English portal of the 4¼-mile-long Severn rail tunnel. As of 2018 the vehicle is still in service, having undergone significant bodywork and mechanical alterations in 2009. It is currently based at Avonmouth. 1998.

Rural Rescue Unit

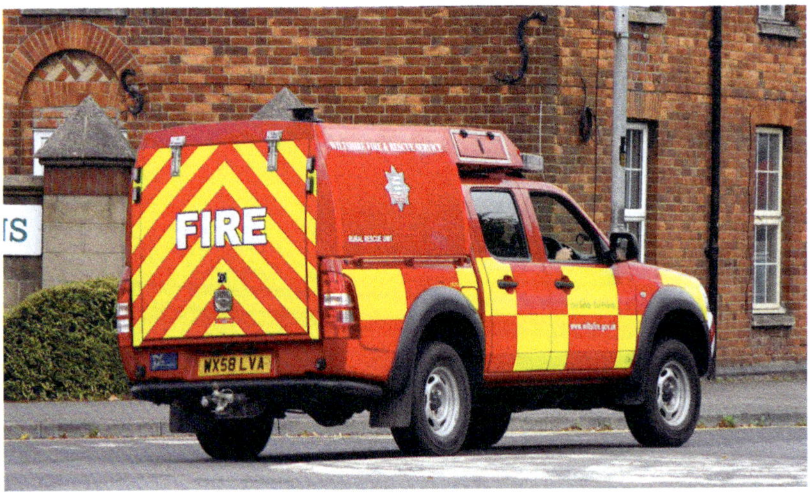

Dorset & Wiltshire Fire & Rescue Service Ford Ranger WX58 LVA, pictured near Warminster, is an ideally suited vehicle for off-road tasks involving animal rescue. It is equipped to tow a two-axle horse box in brigade livery. 2014. (Image: Margaret Boulter)

Water Carriers

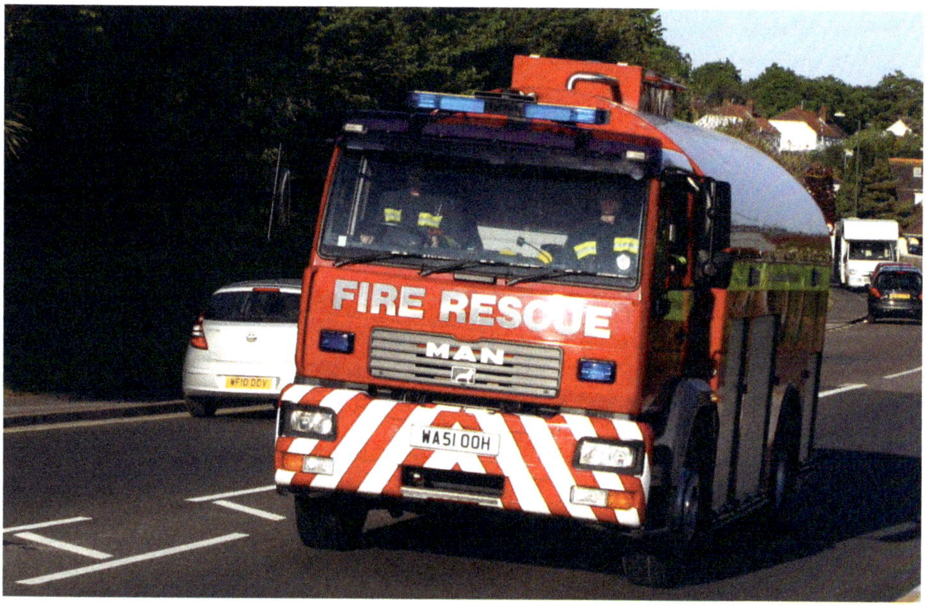

On a hot summer's evening, Torquay fire station's MAN Water Carrier responds on the blues in Newton Road to a fire on wasteland in nearby Kingkerswell. With no hydrants at the location, the appliance was backwards and forwards from the fireground to its nearby home station for water replenishment. This appliance was also able to double as a Foam Carrier. 2011.

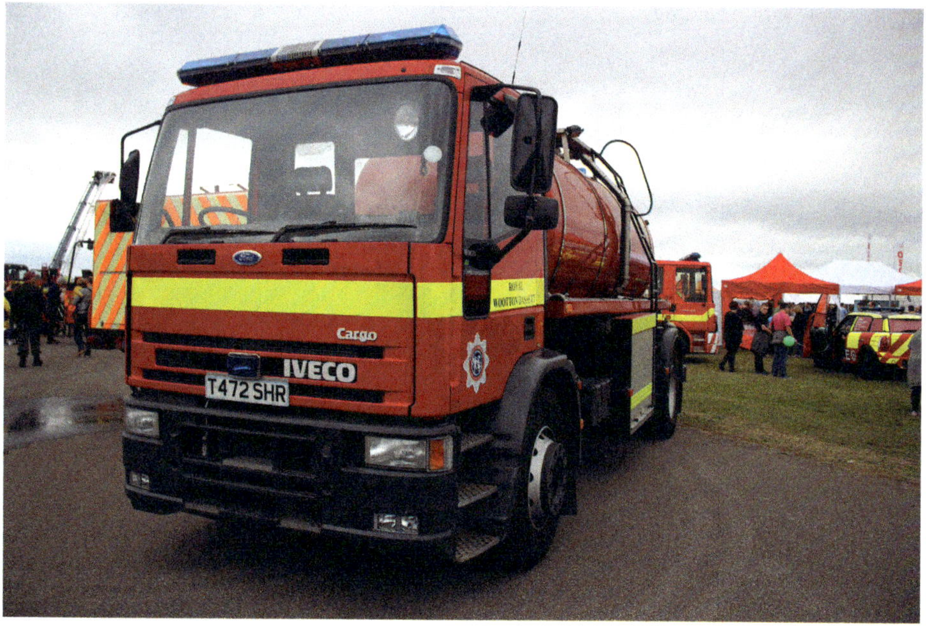

Royal Wootton Bassett's immaculate-looking 1999-registered Iveco Water Carrier T472 SHR is seen at the Kemble 999 Show. 16 September 2018.

Chapter 4

Police

Air Support

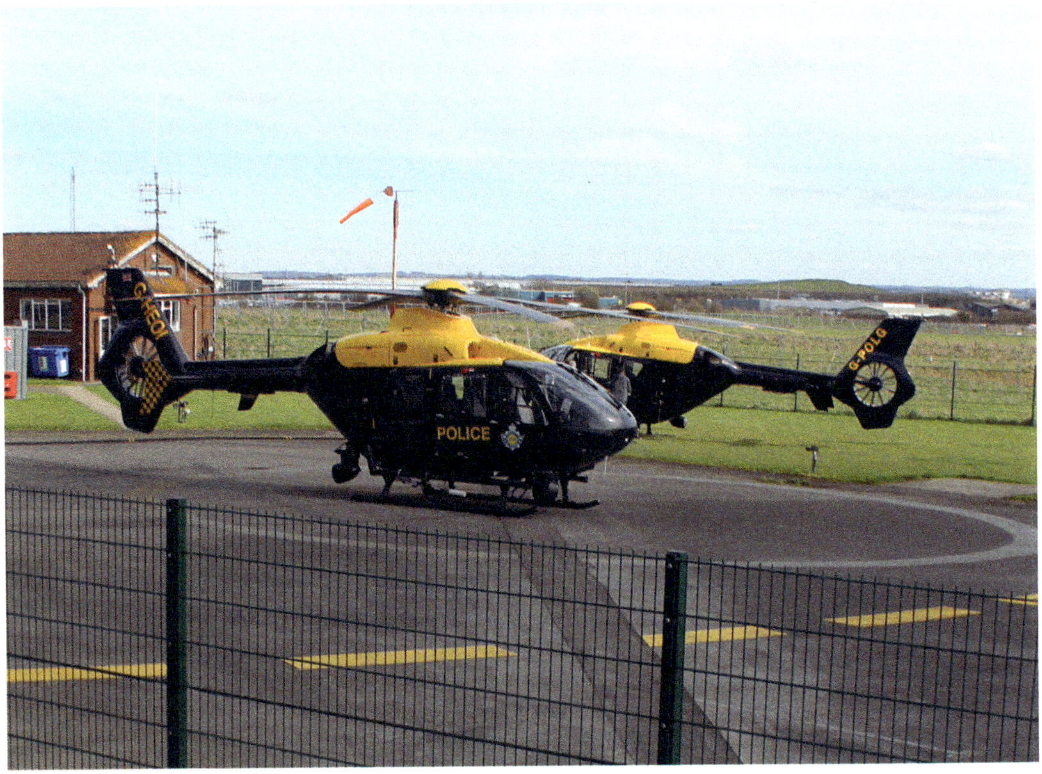

The National Police Air Service (NPAS) Eurocopter, registration G-HEOI, was acting as Filton's regular machine at what is now an archive image – the base moved to Almondsbury in late 2018. Alongside is visiting aircraft G-POLG, which has just landed for refuelling. 5 April 2018.

Area Cars

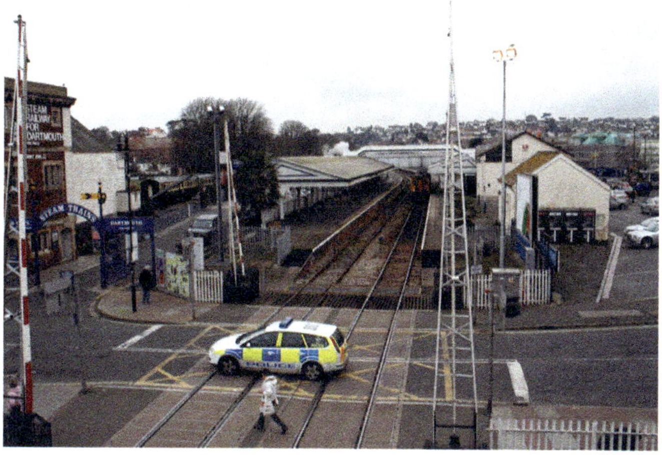

A familiar holiday view is the Network Rail interchange with the Paignton & Dartmouth Steam Railway. A local Ford Focus estate area car is heading down Torbay Road towards Paignton seafront. 2008.

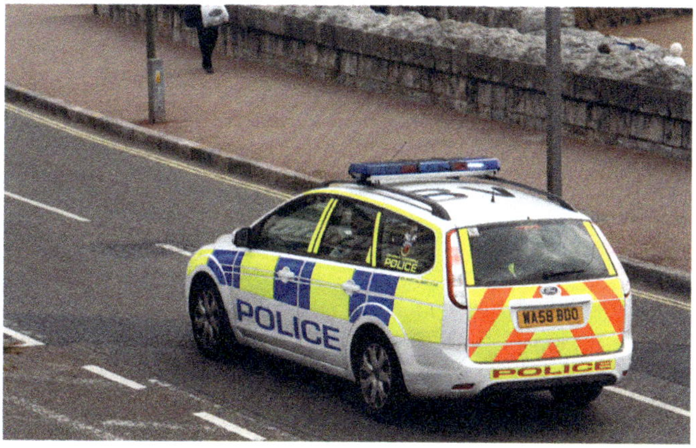

On the seafront at Torquay Ford Focus estate, WA58 BDO is captured making an emergency response towards the town centre. 2010.

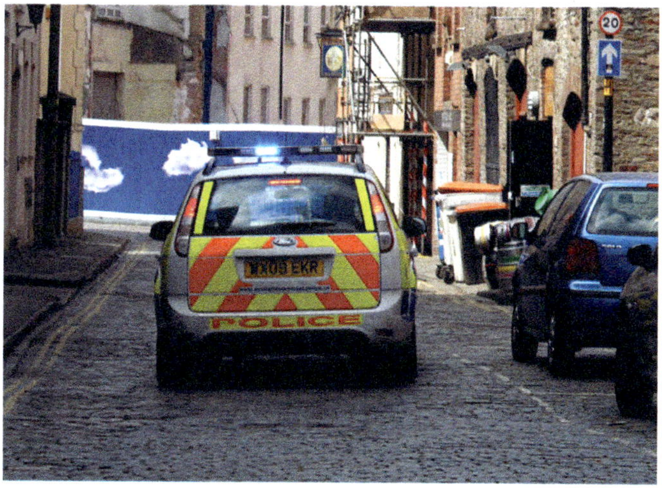

Moving through the old cobbled streets near Queen Square, Bristol, a central area Ford Focus estate quietly edges forward, a silent approach being the order of the day on this occasion, hence no siren in use. 22 November 2012.

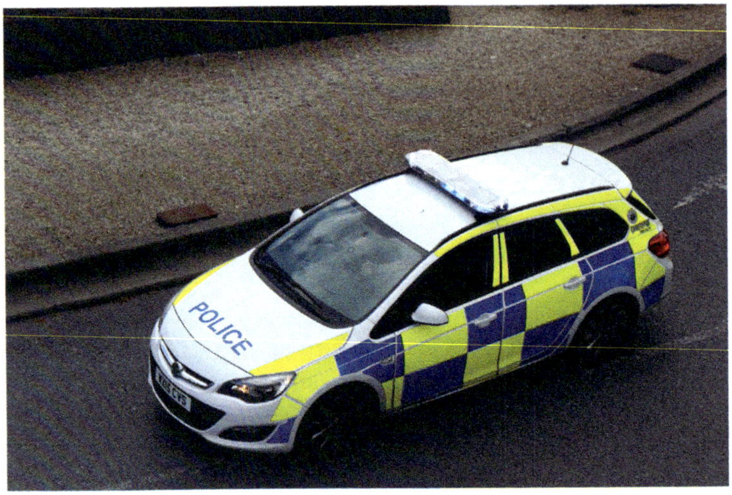

Vauxhall Astra estate WX15 CVS heads around Old Market roundabout for Lawrence Hill in a shot taken from a now demolished footbridge overlooking the roundabout. 4 May 2017.

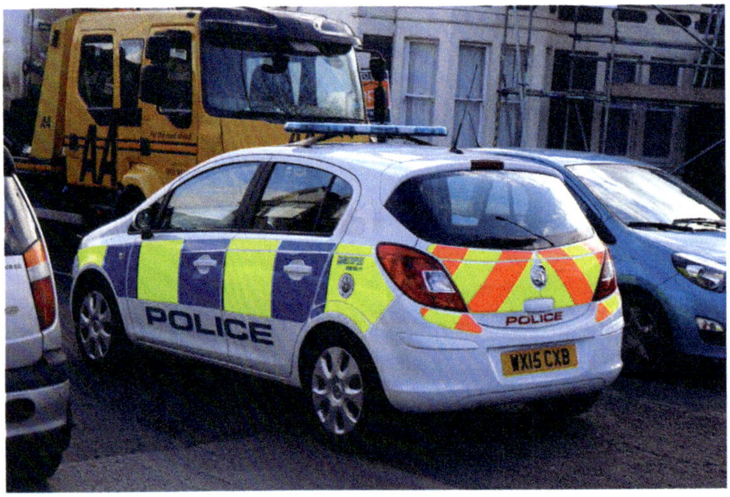

Avon & Somerset have progressively introduced Vauxhall Corsa saloons throughout the force area. WX15 CXB, in pristine exterior condition, is pictured in Horfield. 12 February 2016.

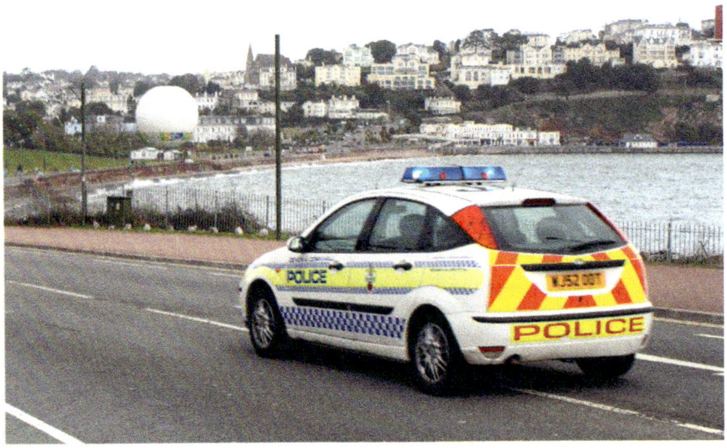

A Devon & Cornwall Ford Focus area car, WJ52 OOT, races towards Torquay at a very high speed in response to an alleged firearms incident. In the distance is the seafront balloon, a tourist attraction over several summers around that period in time. 2010.

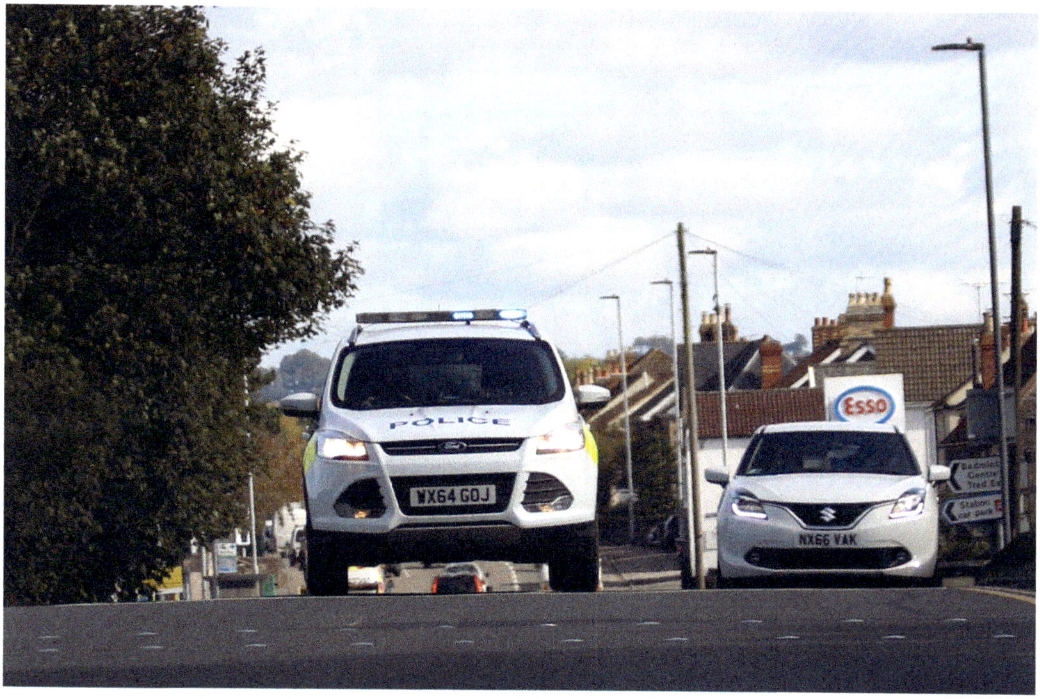

Cresting the Station Road railway bridge at Yate, Chipping Sodbury-based Ford Kuga WX64 GOJ heads on its emergency towards Coalpit Heath. 28 September 2017. (Image: Margaret Boulter)

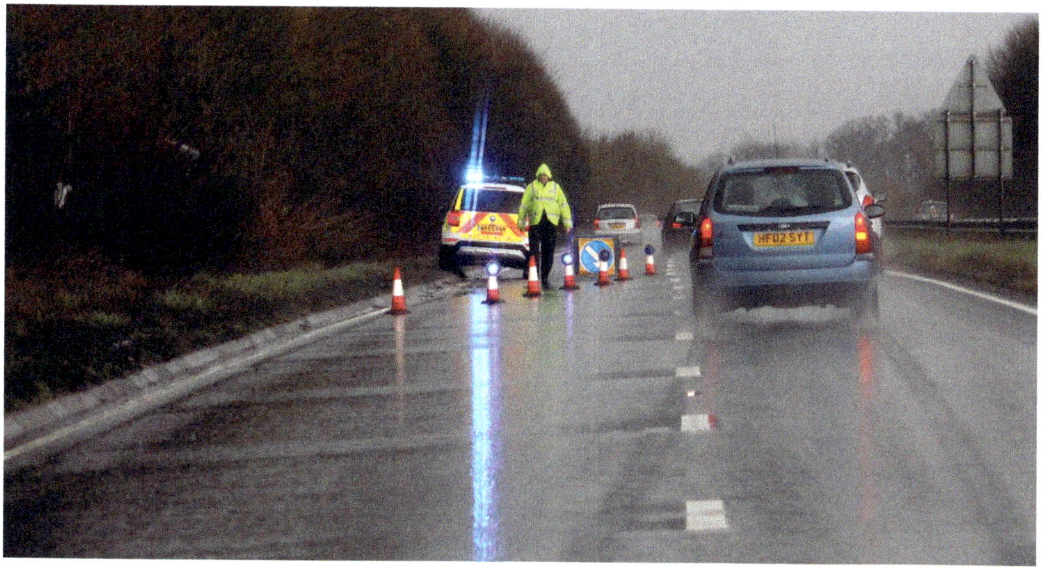

With the infamous Storm Katie brewing (see page 36) and ready to unleash 100-mph winds as well as having already released torrential rain, foul weather was encountered leaving Salisbury on the A36 for Hampshire. A very wet police officer and his Skoda Yeti vehicle on the blues warn of the spot where a private car almost totally hidden in the embankment bushes has left the road. 27 March 2016. (Image: Margaret Boulter)

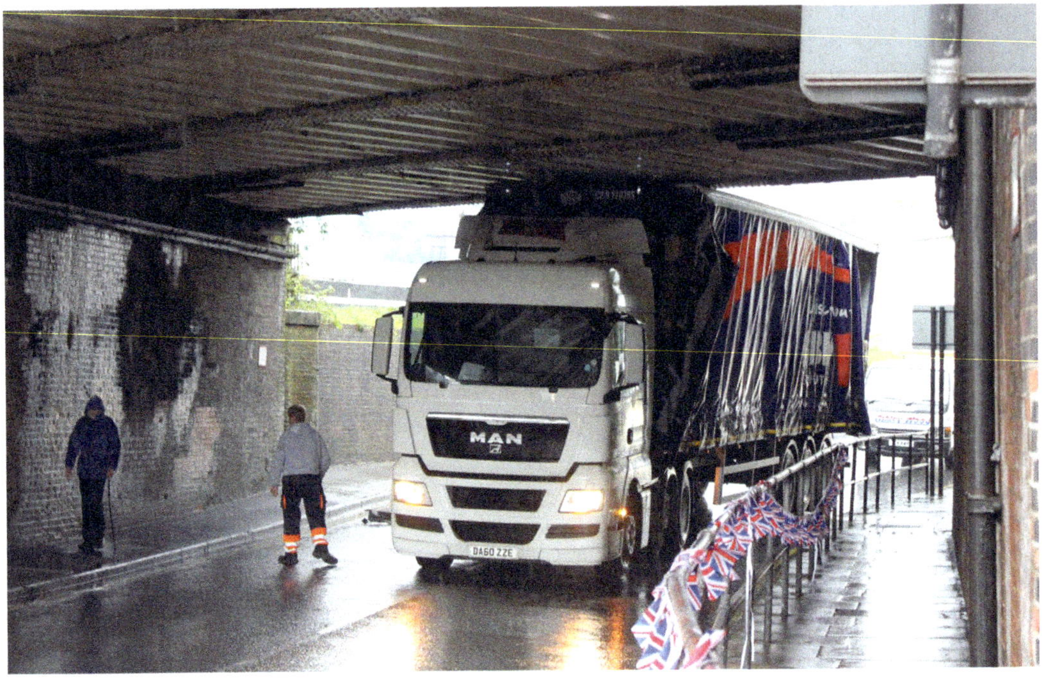

Literally seconds out of his cab, the bewildered driver looks towards the passing pedestrian, perhaps for words of comfort, after striking the Fisherton Street railway bridge just yards outside of Salisbury railway station. With the countdown having started to the arrival of the Royal Train carrying Her Majesty due in the railway station that morning, no doubt the police (who are out of shot just seconds away) will not be lost for words, even if the pedestrian was! 1 May 2012.

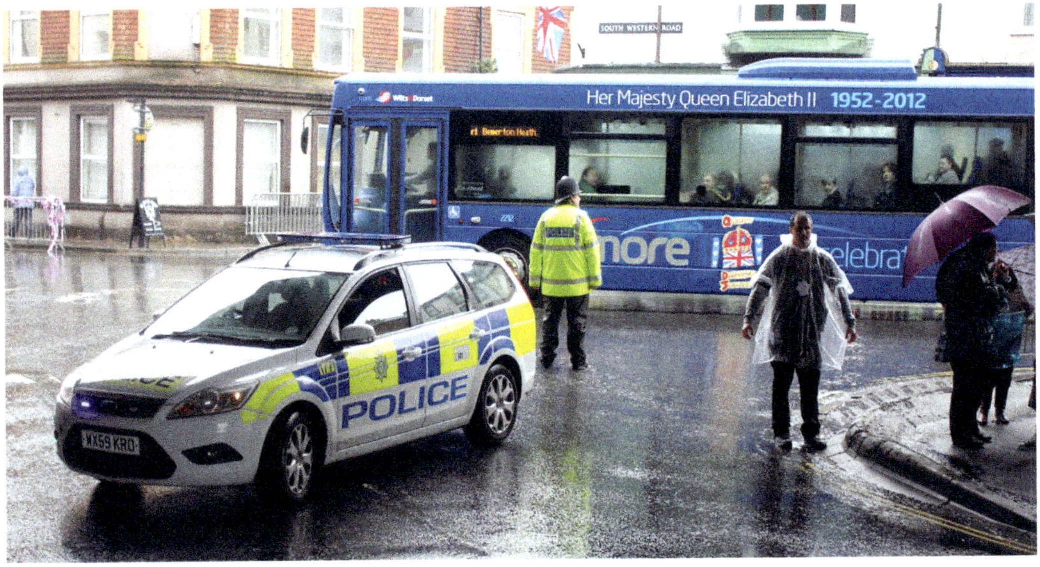

By pure coincidence a passing bus records Her Majesty's historic sixty-year reign. As it does, extra police are now in attendance to take up traffic and crowd control at the bridge strike. 1 May 2012.

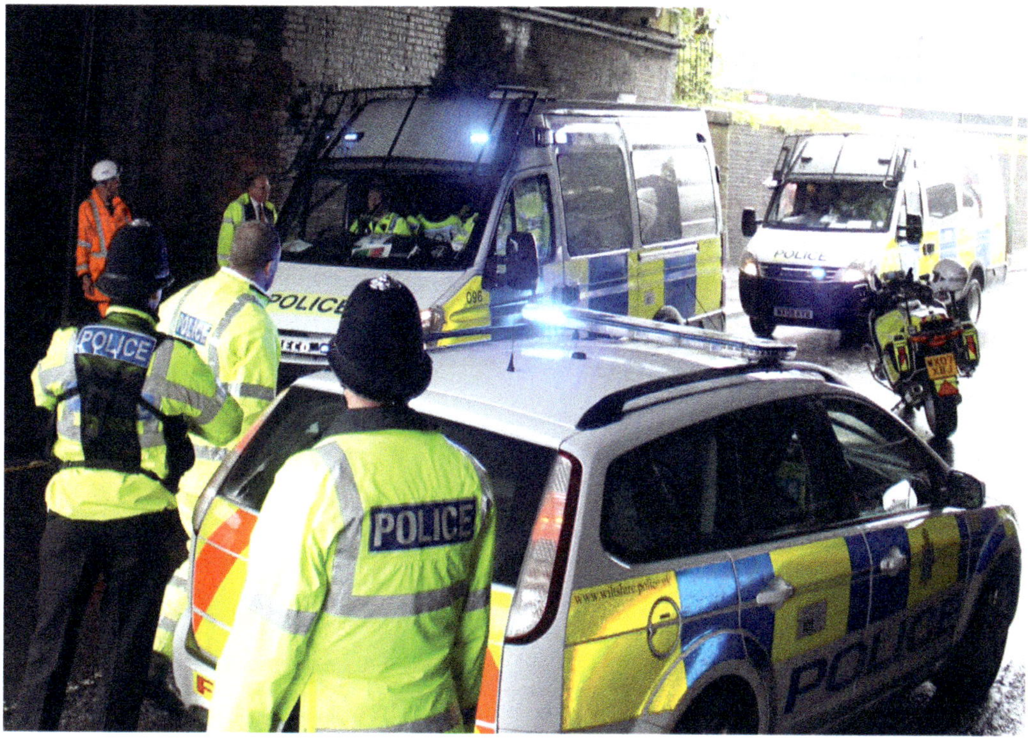

Fortunately Network Rail engineers were almost immediately on scene, the stricken vehicle was reversed a short distance to await a heavy recovery truck's arrival and the bridge was declared safe. With Her Majesty's arrival now less than an hour away, supporting police crews for the historic event are seen traversing Fisherton Street. 1 May 2012.

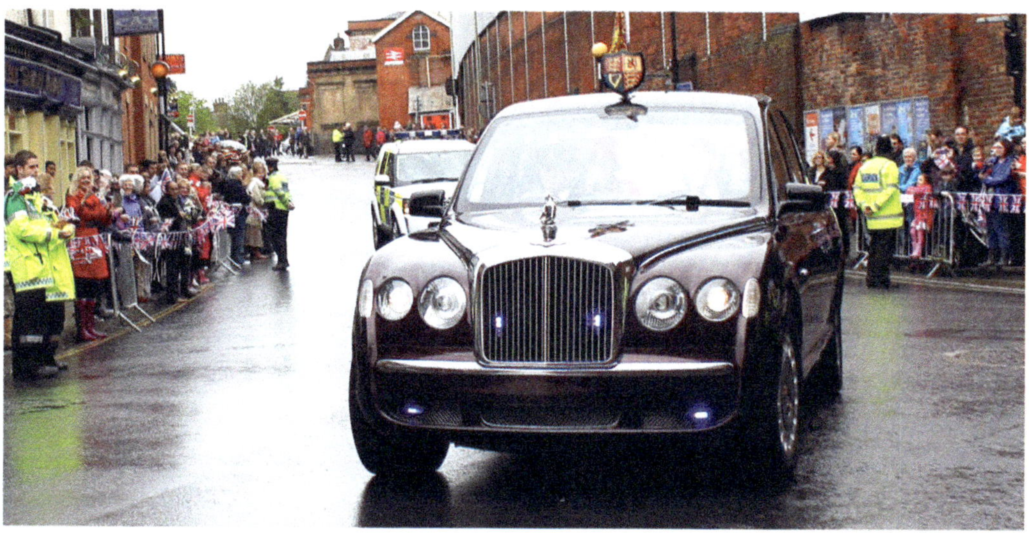

Her Majesty safely in the Royal Car and the torrential rain having eased, her Bentley heads down the incline from the railway station. Vehicles belonging personally to the monarch do not carry registration plates. 1 May 2012.

Armed Response Unit

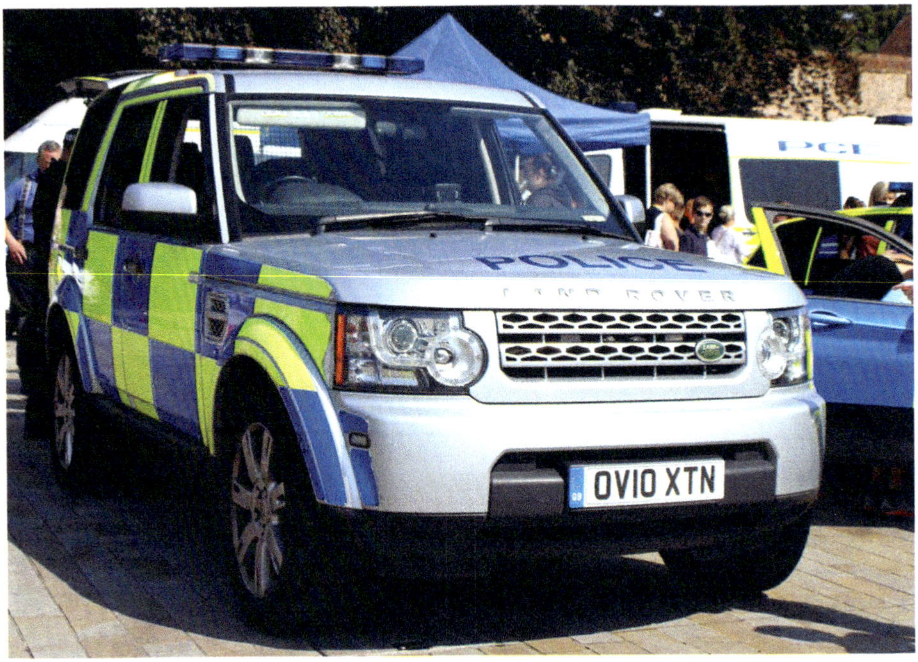

Armed response Land Rover Discovery OV10 XTN, seen on public display at Taunton. 17 August 2015.

Command, Control and Communications

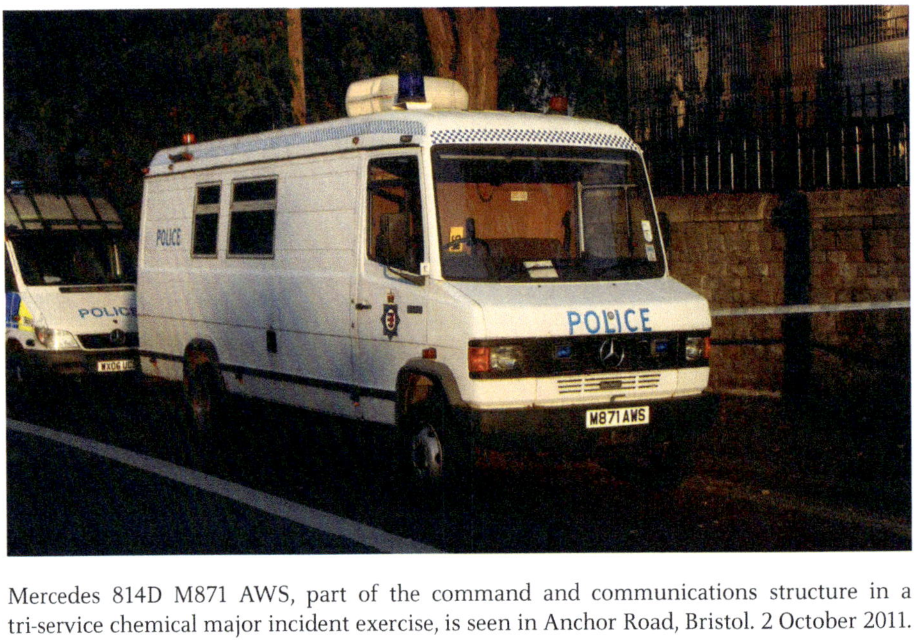

Mercedes 814D M871 AWS, part of the command and communications structure in a tri-service chemical major incident exercise, is seen in Anchor Road, Bristol. 2 October 2011.

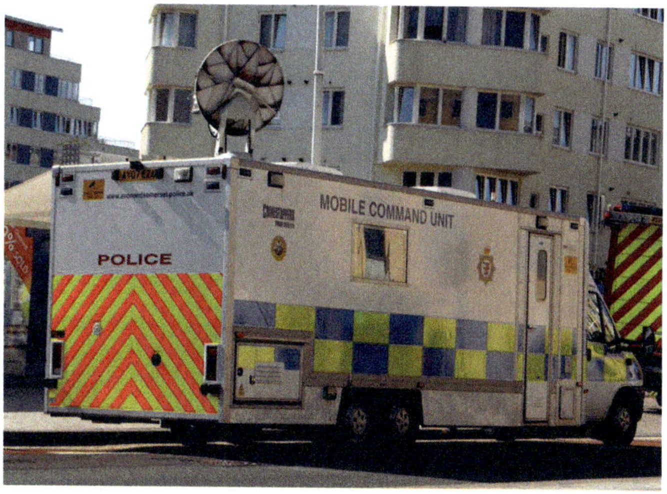

AY07 EZA was another element of the police command at the Anchor Road exercise. 2 October 2011. (Image: Matt Holmes)

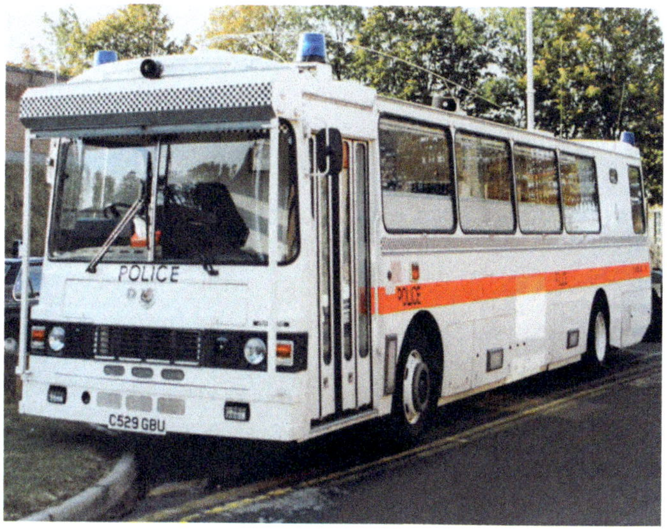

A rare visitor to the Bristol area was a Ministry of Defence Police Command & Communications Unit, one of two similar vehicles. C529 GBU (above) and D658 YCD were deployed on large operations throughout the British mainland in the 1990s, including the latter registered unit at the opening of the massive MOD Procurement Executive complex at Abbey Wood, Filton, by HM the Queen. 1996. (Source unknown)

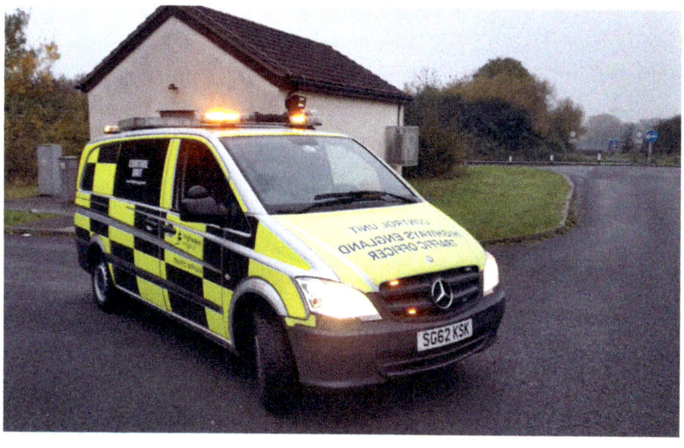

Pictured in South Gloucestershire in experimental markings as a Control Unit, Mercedes Vito SG62 KSK was trialled as a traffic officer's vehicle with Highways England. 29 October 2016. (Image: Matt Holmes)

Community Contact/Neighbourhood Policing

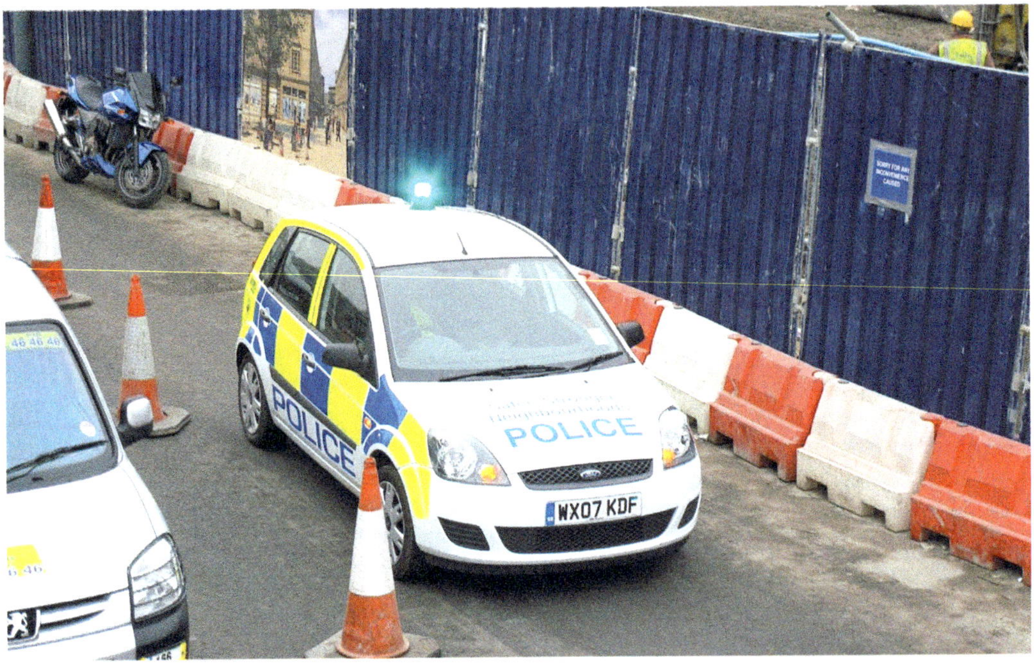

A police community support officer's Ford Fiesta pictured in Bath with a magnetic portable blue light displayed on the roof. 2007.

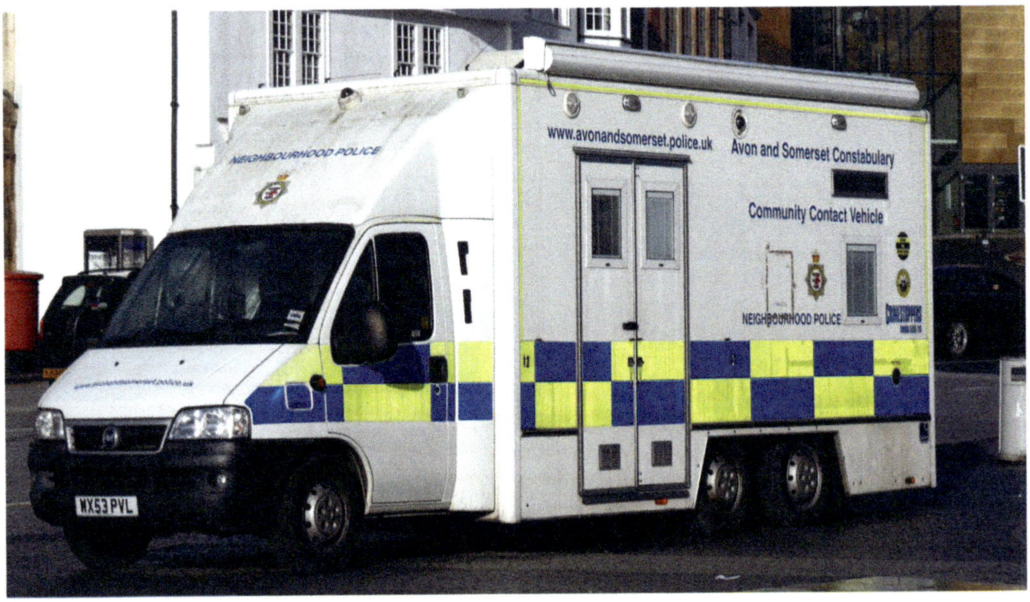

Parked and unattended in Bristol city centre, this vehicle had no doubt been manned until the early hours, large crowds frequenting the nearby bars and clubs being a regular feature of weekends in the city's harbourside and central area. Believed to be 2012.

Dog Units

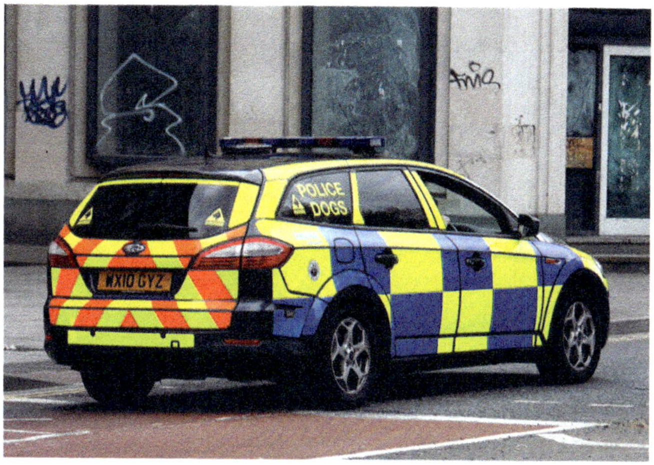

Previously this Bristol-based vehicle was unmarked. Subsequently, it was converted to battenburg livery while retaining the dark-coloured base paintwork. 25 April 2015.

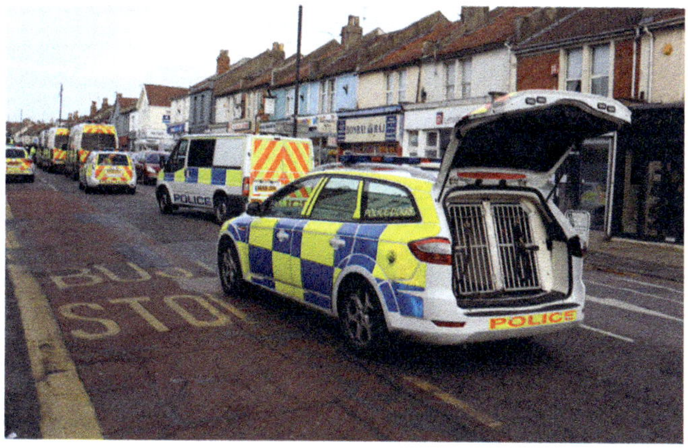

A heavy police contingent keeps a watchful eye on football supporters heading towards the Bristol Rovers football ground in nearby Filton Avenue. The Mondeo dog van is ready for immediate deployment as it slowly edges up Gloucester Road towards the Memorial Stadium. 23 January 2016.

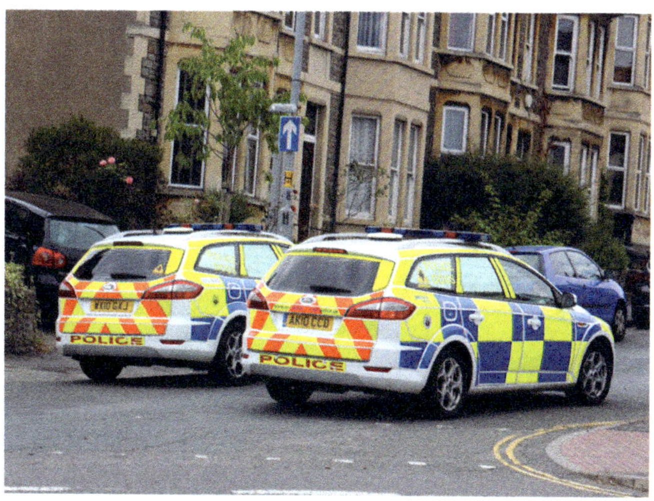

Two Mondeo dog van units side by side block the entrance into Wellington Hill, Horfield, Bristol, pending further instructions from their control, who are monitoring the movement of the early season football crowd. 14 August 2016.

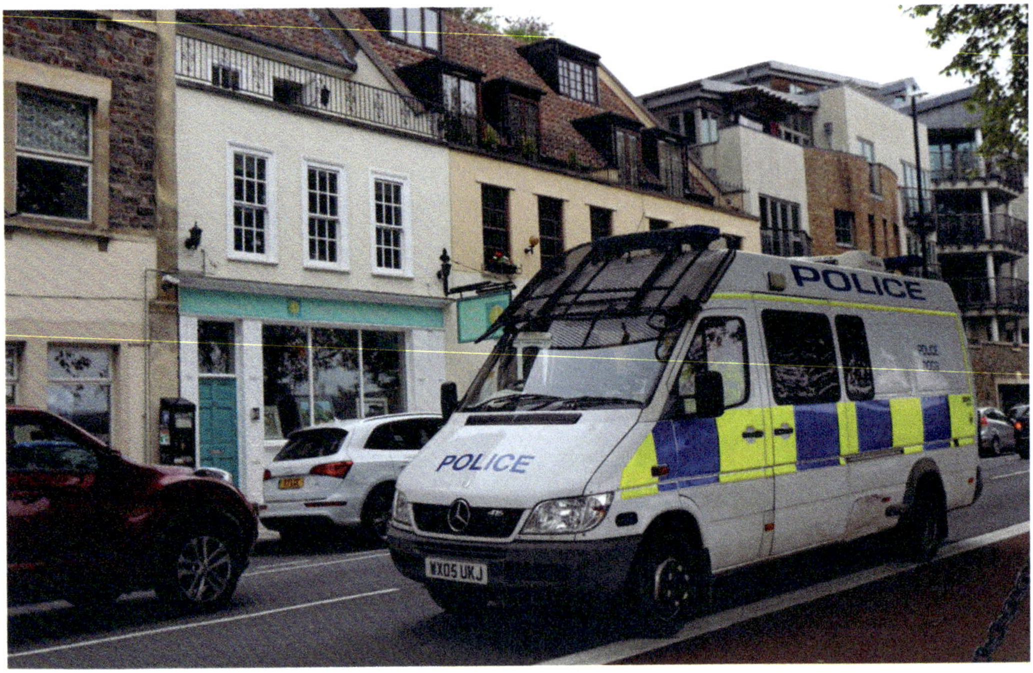

Capable of comfortably housing six animals, a Mercedes Sprinter dog van makes its way down Hotwell Road, Bristol. Demonstrators at a public order incident are within seconds of reaching this spot. However, the rapid deployment of three dogs, along with four police horses and public order trained personnel already in situ, soon prevented the crowd from advancing further. 4 June 2016.

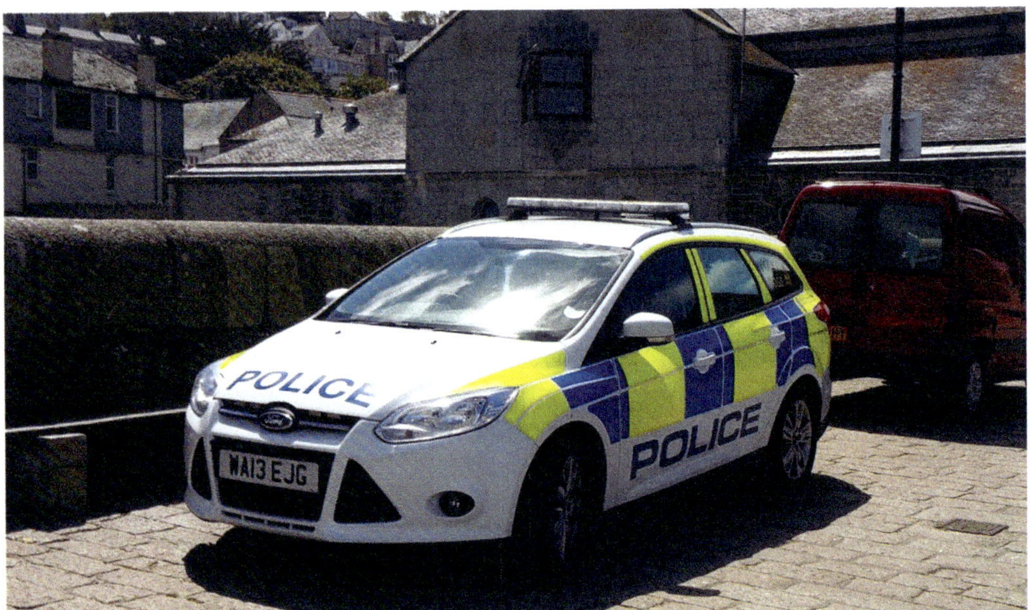

Cornwall-based Ford Focus estate police dog unit WA13 EJG is pictured in the beautiful town of St Ives. May 2016. (Image: Matt Holmes)

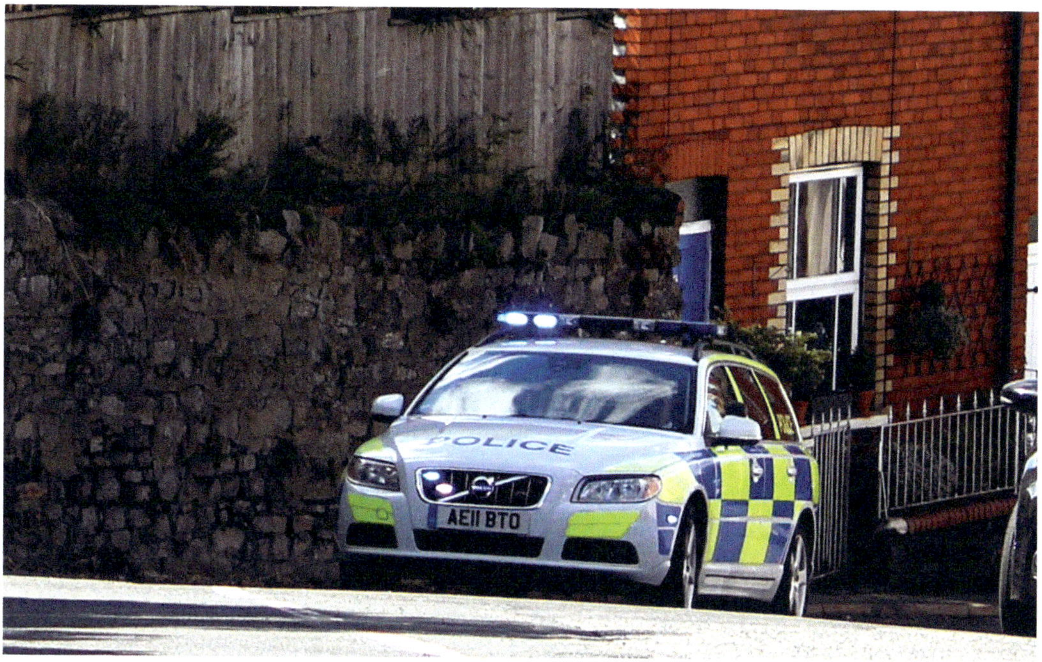

On the blues and twos, Volvo estate AE11 BTO climbs the very steep Waters Lane, Westbury-on-Trym, Bristol. 29 April 2015.

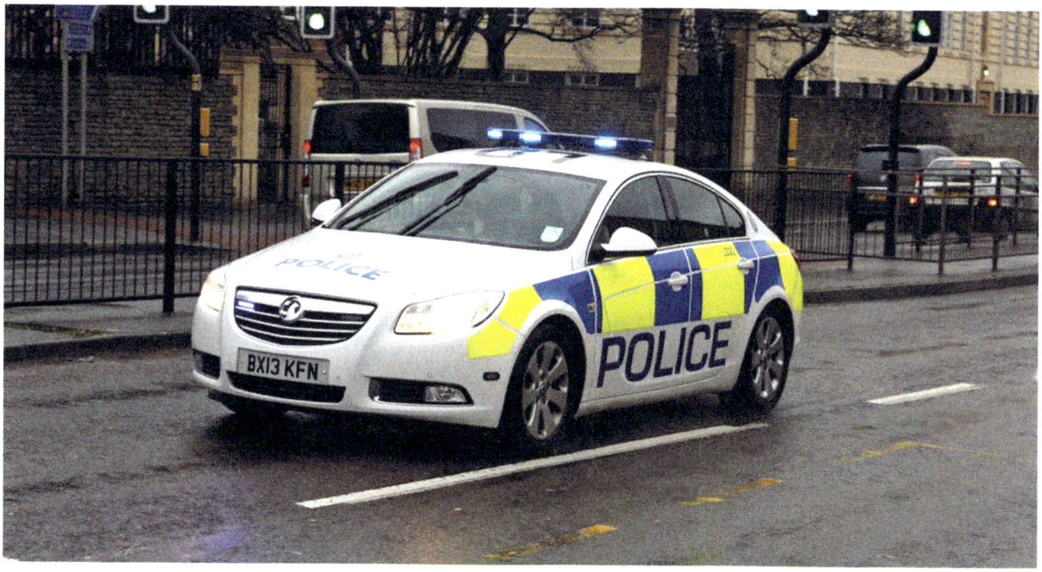

It is probable that this West Midlands Police VX Insignia saloon was engaged in advanced driver training, with long distances on the blue light and siren being normal for drivers undergoing rigorous training and assessment. The vehicle is seen on the A38 at Filton as it enters Bristol. 27 January 2016.

Fleet Support/Recovery

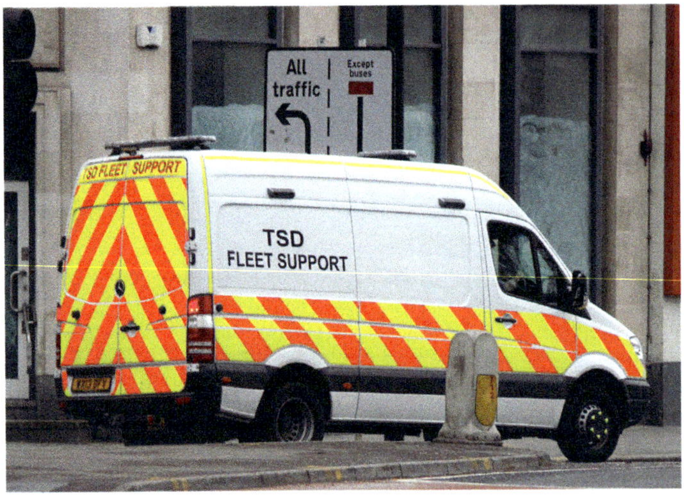

No emergency service can function effectively without the first-class support of its fleet engineering department. One of Avon & Somerset Police Mercedes fleet support vehicles, WX13 DFV, is pictured in Bristol city centre. 28 February 2015.

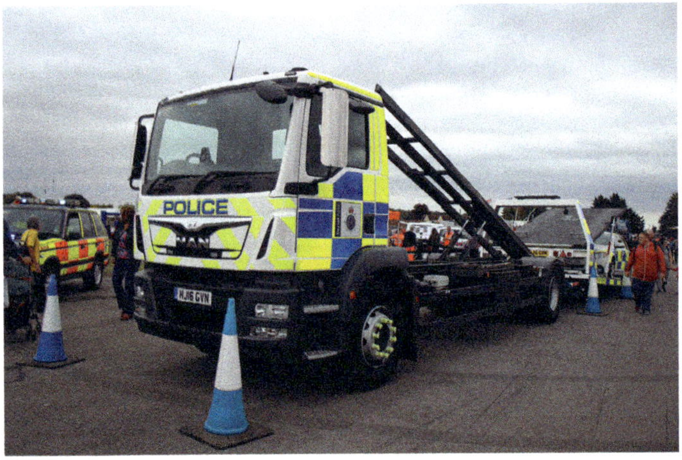

On display at the Kemble 999 Show was this smart-looking Dorset Police MAN Recovery Vehicle, HJ16 GVN. 16 September 2018.

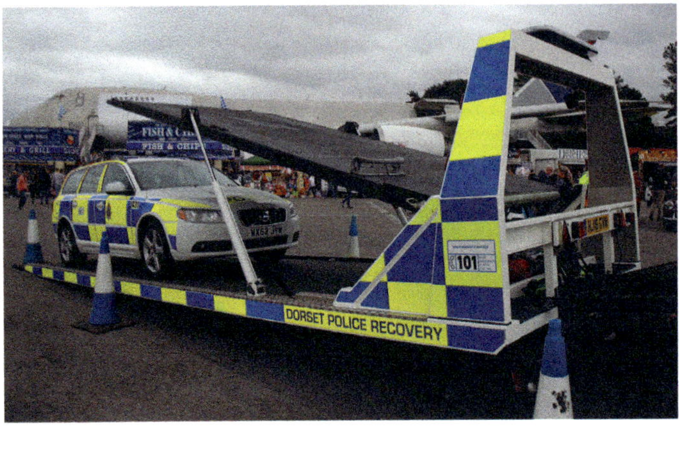

Positioned on the lower deck of the tilting trailer was Wiltshire Police traffic Volvo estate WX62 JYW.

Land Rover

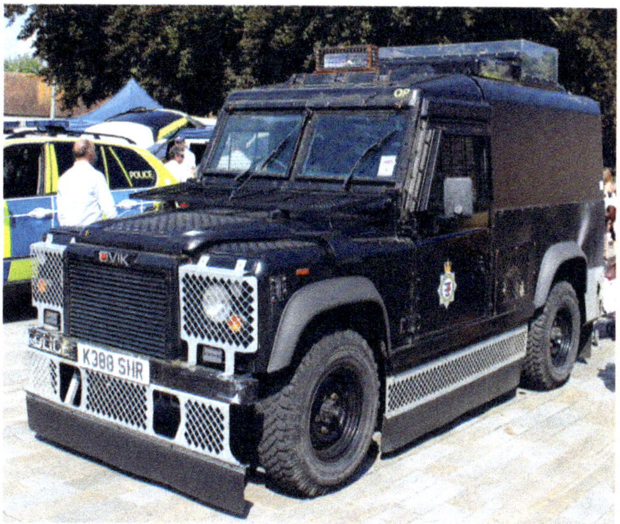

An austere-looking Land Rover is pictured on display in Taunton. The protection is necessary for the more robust tasks it may be called upon to perform. 17 August 2015.

Mounted Section

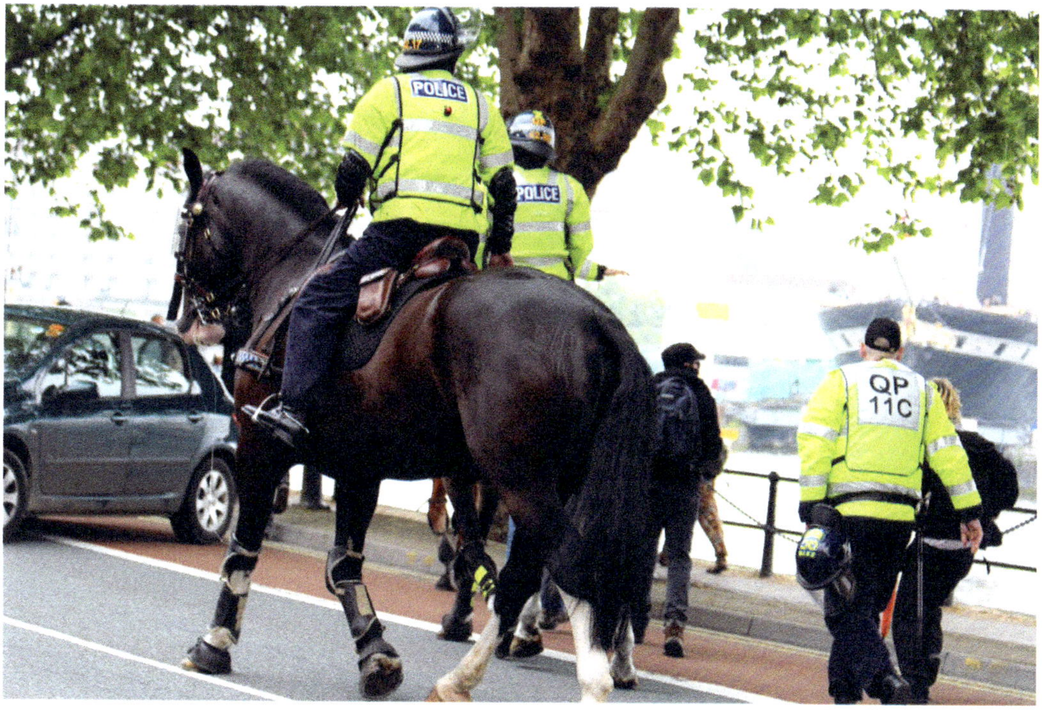

The mere presence of a mighty horse is sufficient to ensure compliance from most people! With Brunel's iconic SS *Great Britain* in the background, two mounted officers and a colleague on foot gently encourage innocent pedestrians, motorists and others perhaps not so well intentioned to turn around and head away from trouble occurring further back down the road. 4 June 2016.

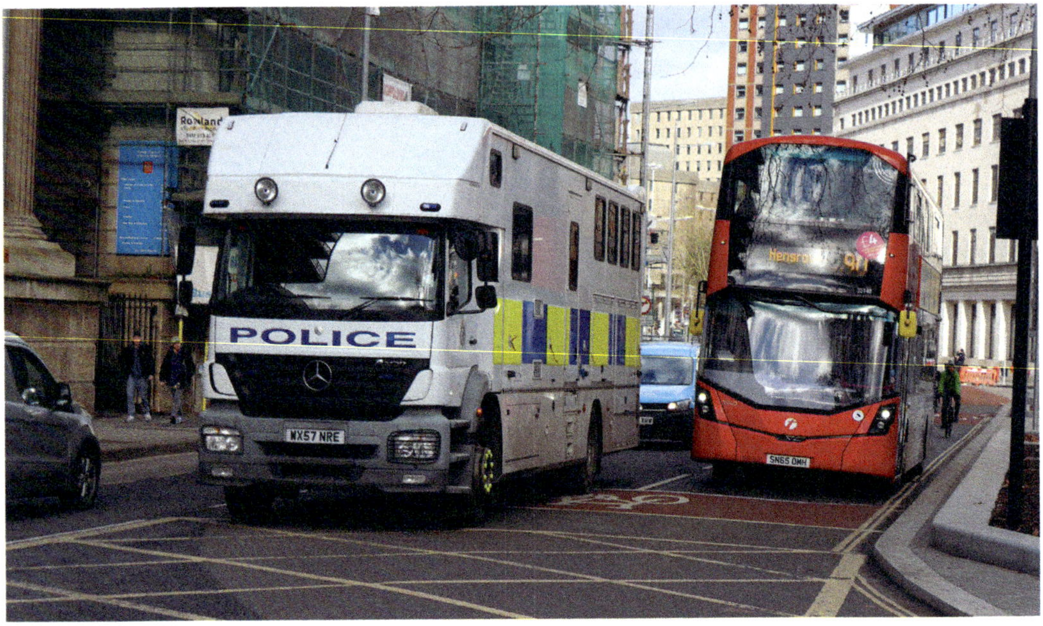

Mercedes horsebox WX57 NRE, one of a matching pair in the force, makes its way across Bristol city centre. 9 February 2018.

Public Order Support Units

Images from what was Bristol's biggest public order deployment for four years appear in the next shots, taken on 4 June 2016, with assistance to Avon & Somerset being provided by Devon & Cornwall, Dorset, Welsh and Wiltshire public order trained personnel. Three dog handlers, eight mounted officers and four roads policing motorcycle personnel were very much part of this impressive and successful deployment to keep the citizens of Bristol safe, to keep rival factions separated and to minimise damage.

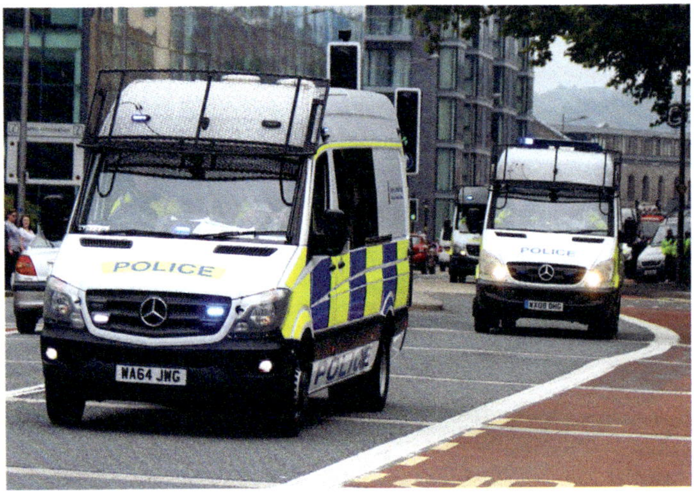

Officers were soon into action! Well before lunchtime a public order support unit of three serials raced up Anchor Road towards the city centre. The leading serial are Devon & Cornwall officers and the second vehicle is from Avon & Somerset.

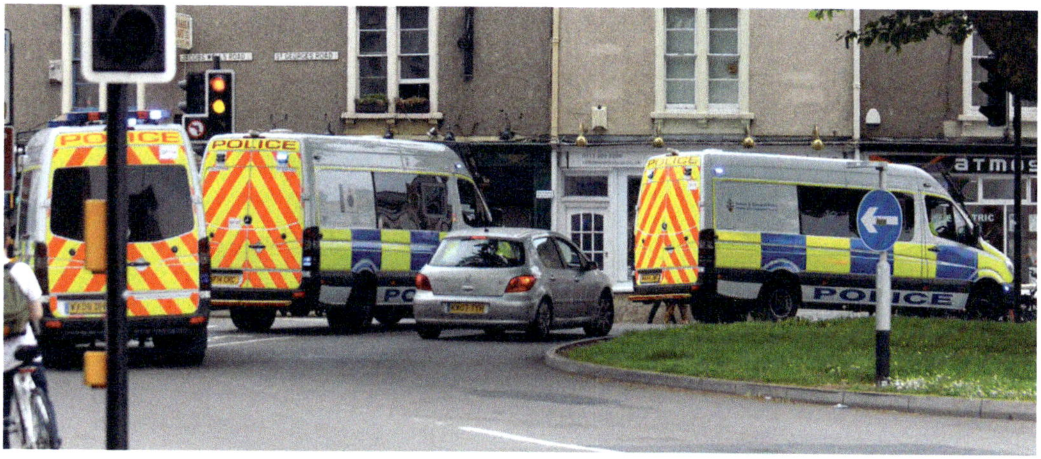

Captured on film is the remarkable sight of a three-vehicle Support Unit, comprising vehicles from Devon & Cornwall (leading), Dorset (middle) and Avon & Somerset Constabulary, all on the blues in central Bristol.

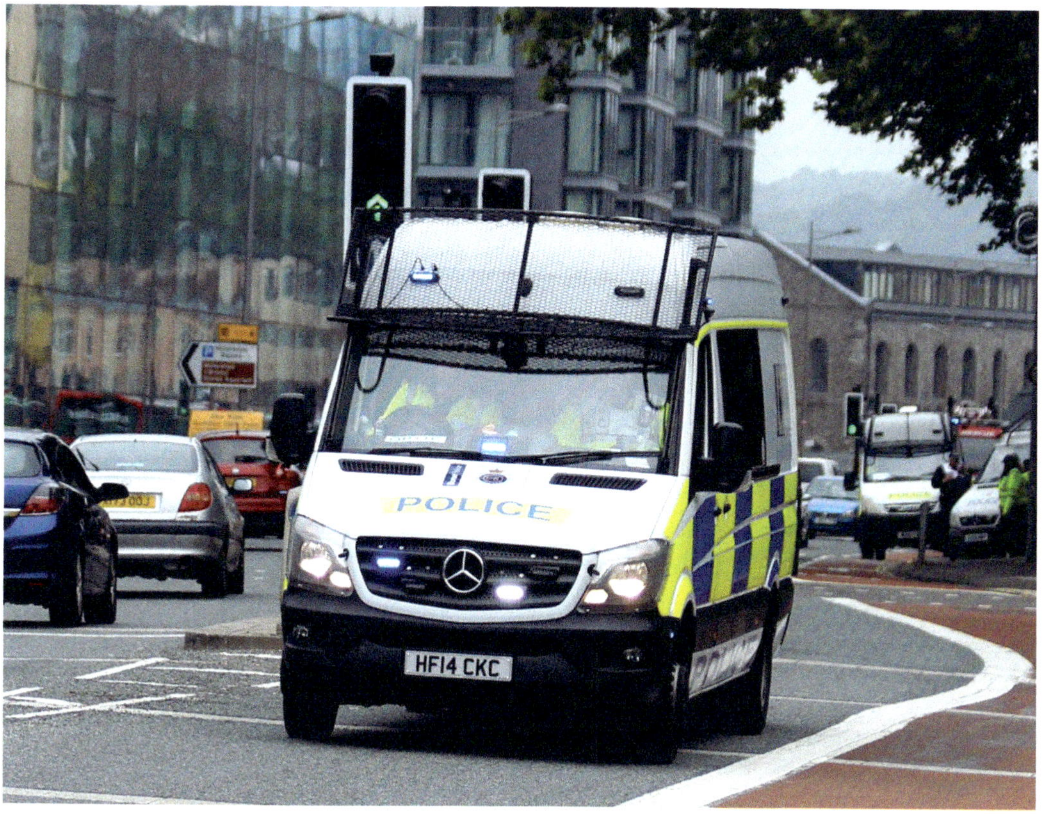

A contingent of Dorset officers head on the blues and twos into central Bristol in a fast-flowing situation involving three rival political groups, not all of whose intentions were thought to be peaceful. Other public order units in the background in Anchor Road are dealing with a minor incident, as is the fire service.

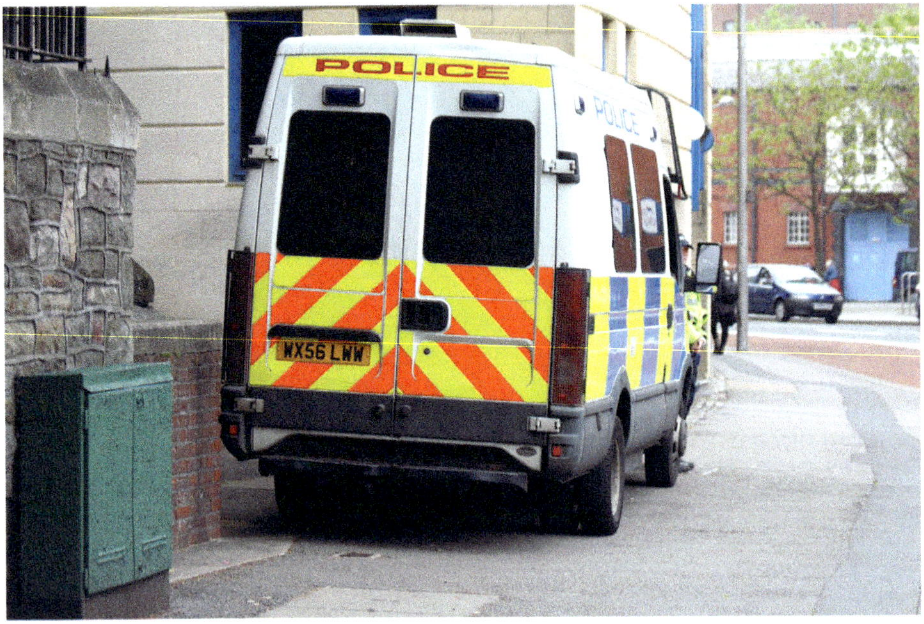

A Wiltshire vehicle is strategically positioned, its crew ready to use any one of a number of routes giving access on foot to likely flash points.

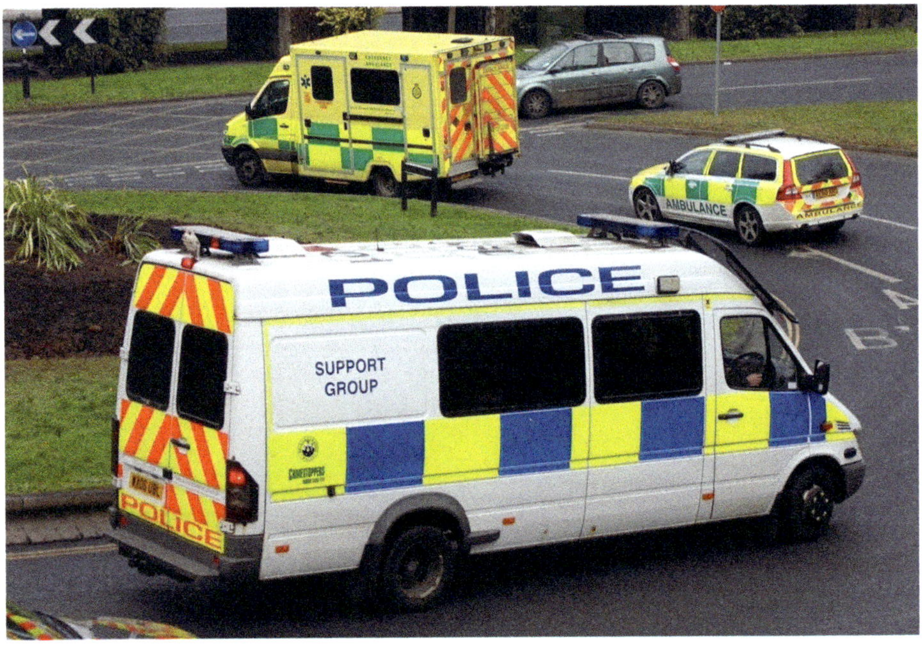

A much quieter scene in Bath. The emergency ambulance appears to be VX58 CDE, followed by Great Western Ambulance Service Volvo estate paramedic car AE60 ARO. Police Mercedes Sprinter WX06 UBL brings up the rear of these three emergency vehicles, which are all travelling at normal road speed at the foot of the A367 Wells Road. 12 February 2012.

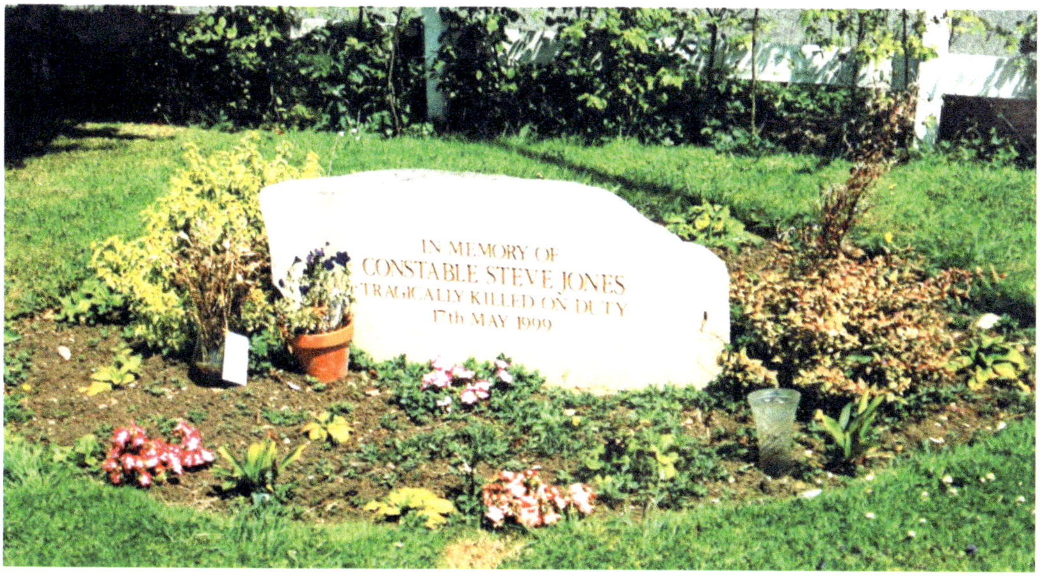
IN MEMORY OF
CONSTABLE STEVE JONES
TRAGICALLY KILLED ON DUTY
17th MAY 1999

Sadly, road traffic collisions are not confined to the general public, with a member of the emergency services occasionally losing their life. This poignant memorial is in the grounds of Almondsbury traffic base, near Bristol. Constable Steve Jones lost his life deploying a stinger to the carriageway of the nearby M4 on 17 May 1999 when he was struck by the suspect vehicle he was attempting to stop. July 2001.

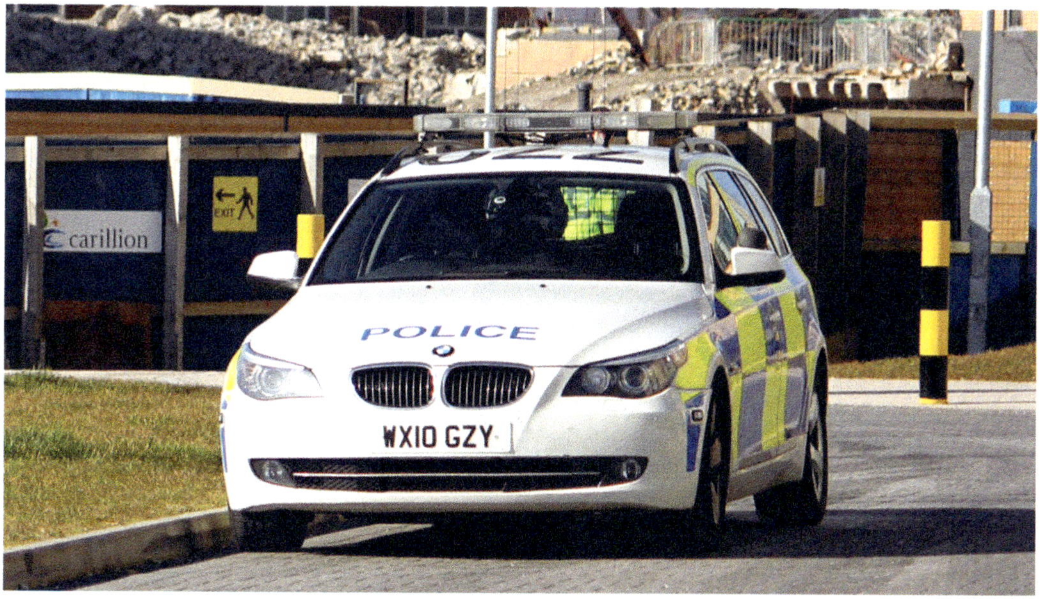
carillion
EXIT
POLICE
WX10 GZY

Typical of most force's roads policing fleet is this BMW 530d tourer, WX10 GZY. Planned building demolition of the old Southmead Hospital makes an unusual background to this image. 10 March 2015.

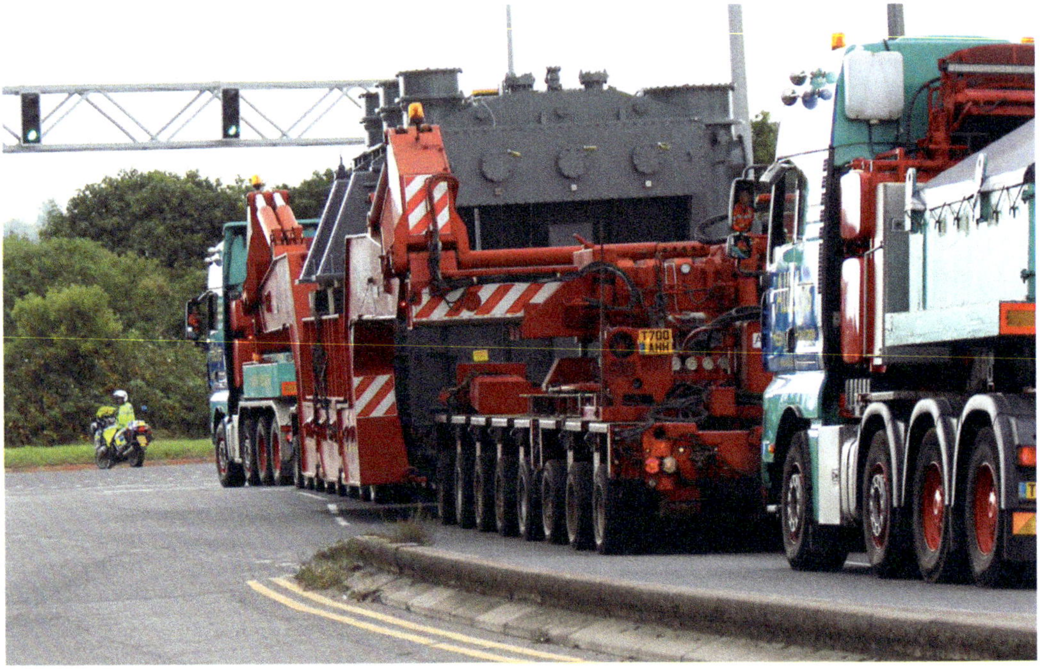

Very much part of a roads policing response are motorcycle officers. In this instance one of several motorcyclists assisting fellow traffic officers in cars can be seen on the approach to the M5 (N) at Junction 18 as the combined police team escort an abnormal load conveying an electrical generator away from Avonmouth Docks. 25 July 2016.

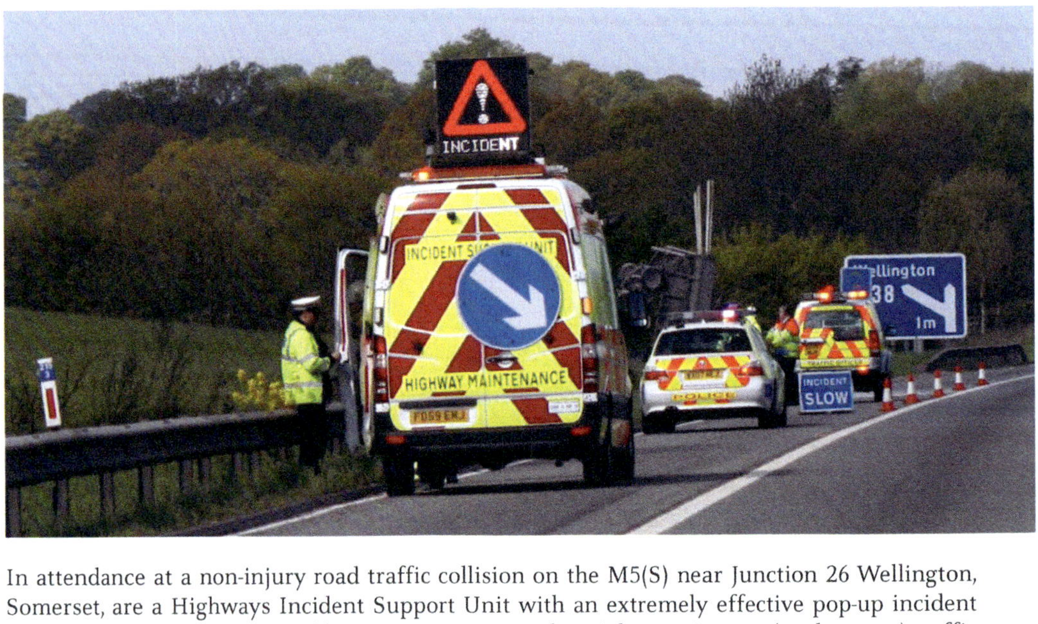

In attendance at a non-injury road traffic collision on the M5(S) near Junction 26 Wellington, Somerset, are a Highways Incident Support Unit with an extremely effective pop-up incident warning sign, police BMW traffic car WX07 MLZ and a Highways Agency (as then was) traffic officer's vehicle. The wreckage of a jack-knifed trailer can be seen in an adjoining field. 2010. (Image: Margaret Boulter)

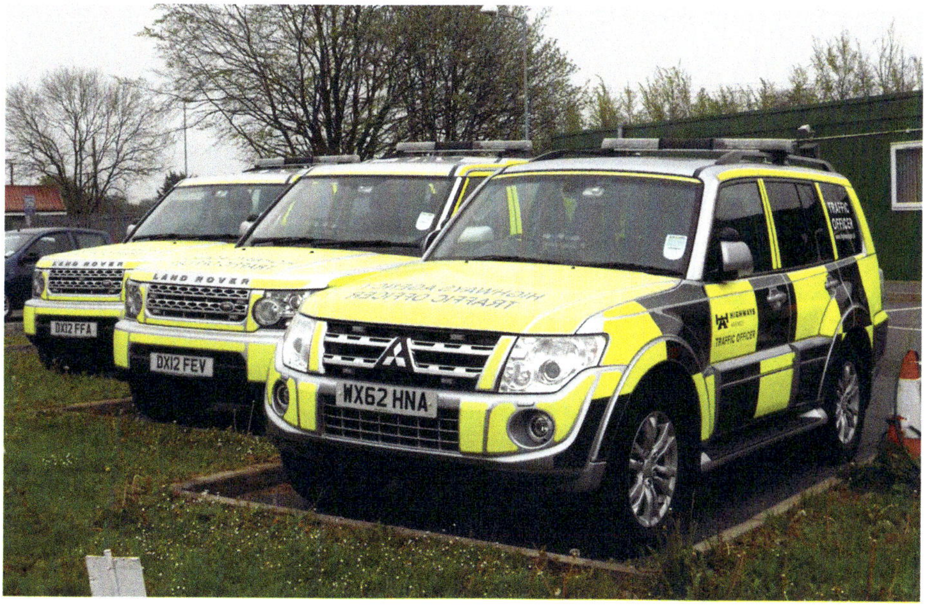

Officers from Highways England (formerly the Highways Agency) perform a vital role helping roads policing officers from local constabularies deployed on the region's motorways and principal 'A' class roads in protecting the scene and restoring normality to traffic flows following an incident. This trio of units are seen north of the region at their M4 Chippenham base. 2013. (Image: Matt Holmes)

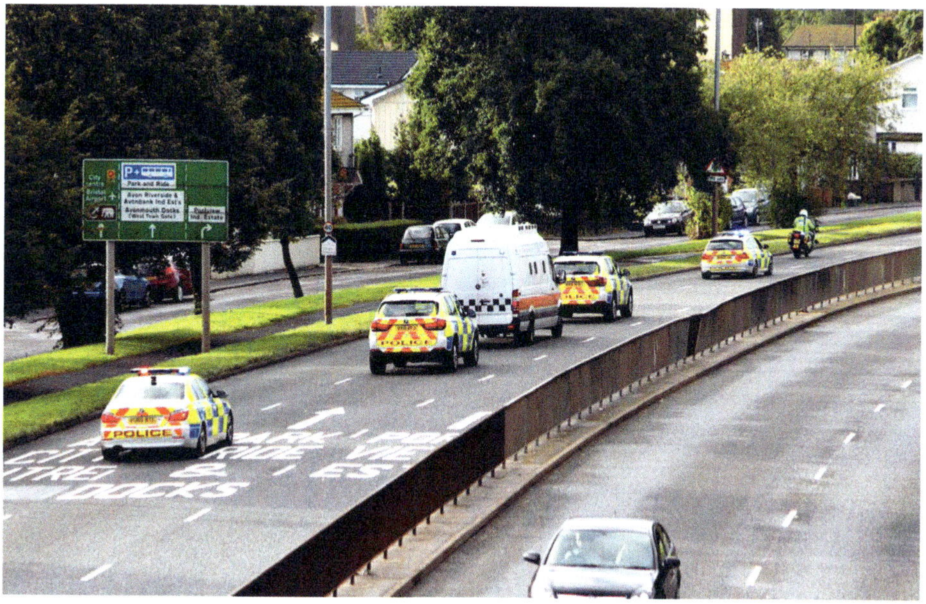

A fast-moving, heavily protected high-security prisoner convoy, all on the blue light with sirens activated, makes its way to Bristol Crown Court from the M5(S) at Avonmouth. Having already gone ahead, further motorcyclists will have shut down side roads to enable the convoy to continue its close escort high-speed run. 24 September 2015.

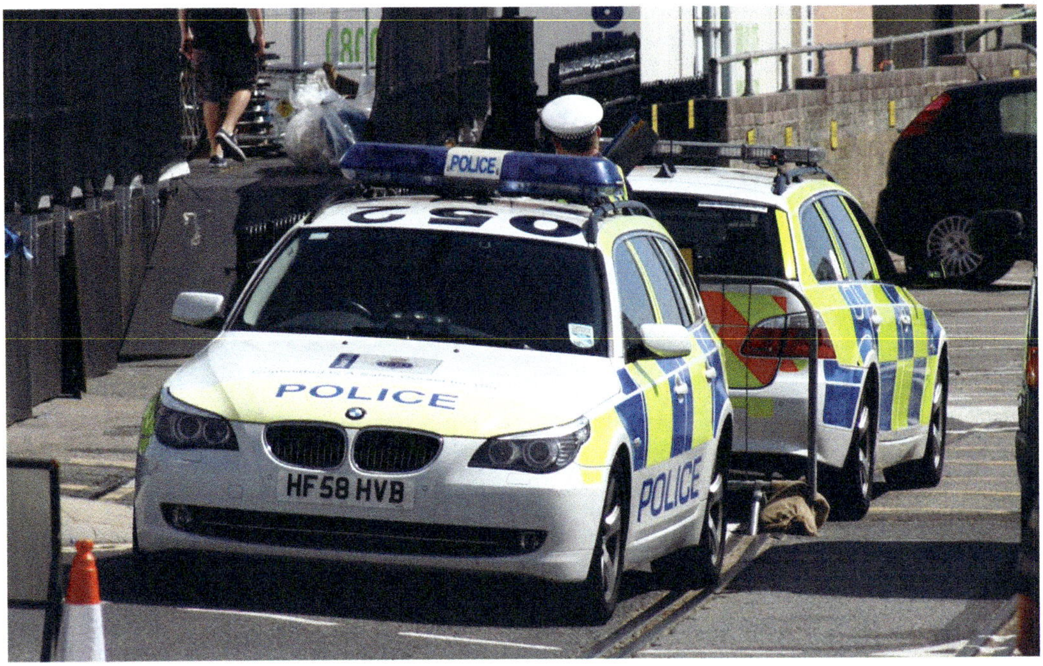

Dorset Police BMW 530d tourer HF58 HVB is pictured in Weymouth as part of the Olympic Games security effort. Sailing events were based off the Dorset coastline. Summer 2012. (Image: Matt Holmes)

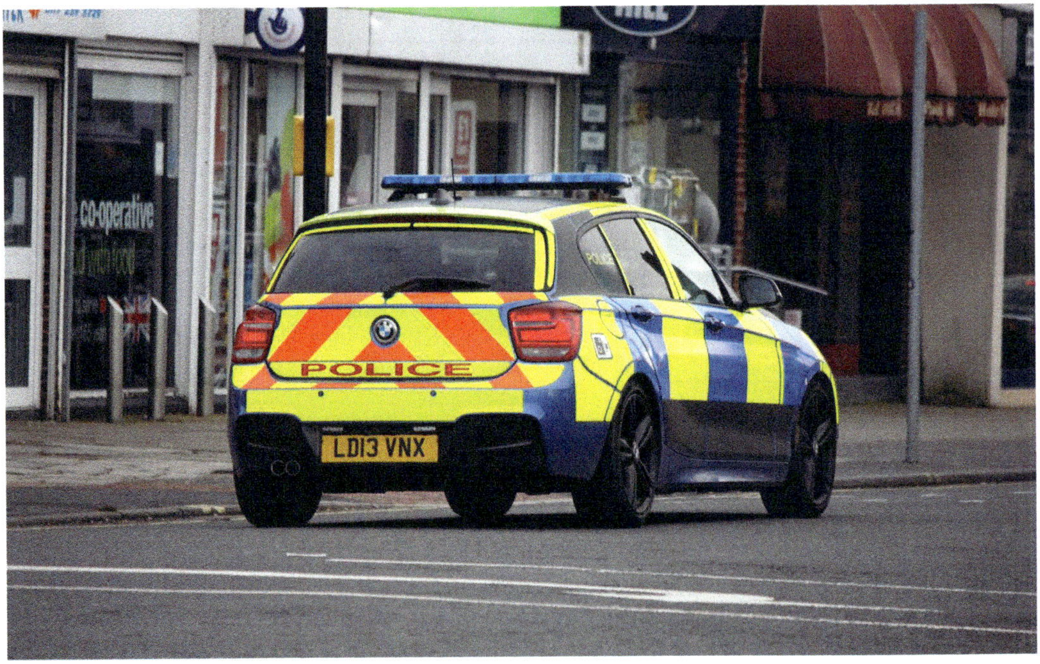

BMW 1 series LD13 VNX is pictured on the A38 Filton Road as it heads towards central Bristol. 26 February 2015. (Image: Margaret Boulter)

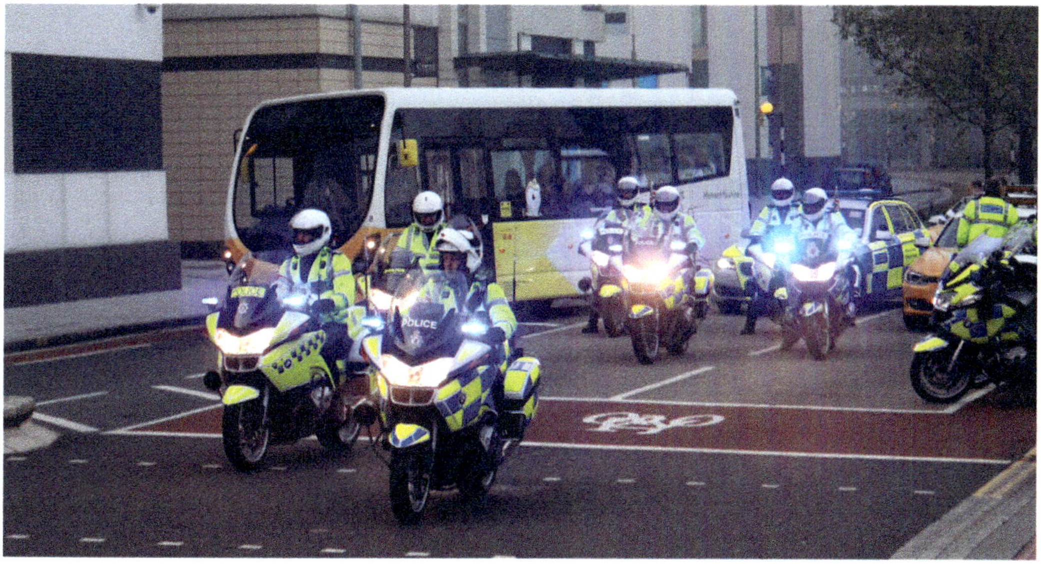

A very early start on Day 5 (of seventy days across the UK) led to this 0550 hours image taken at Canons Way, Bristol, in the morning mist as an element of the Olympic Torch Relay escort motorcyclists headed out. They formed the advance party for the day's first batch of runners, who would shortly follow on their individual 300-metre sections bearing the lit torch. 23 May 2012.

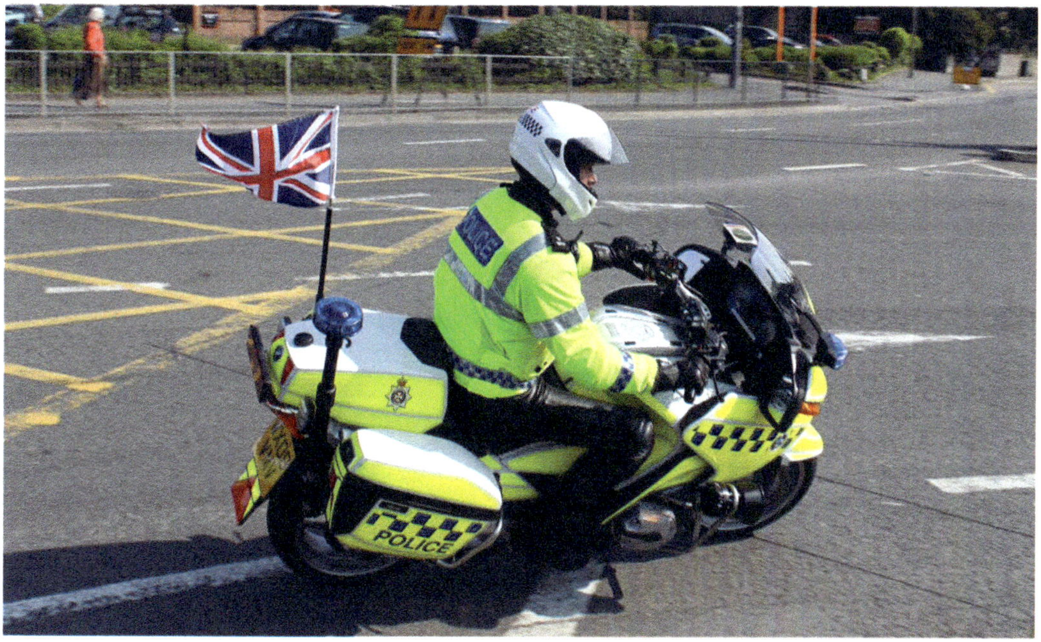

A Wiltshire motorcyclist proudly displaying the Union Flag negotiates Filton roundabout, South Gloucestershire. His machine was part of the huge police escort accompanying the Olympic Torch Relay. With torch bearing duties in the Bristol area now complete, the considerable entourage is about to make its way by road towards Chippenham, where the next relay stages on foot will recommence. 23 May 2012.

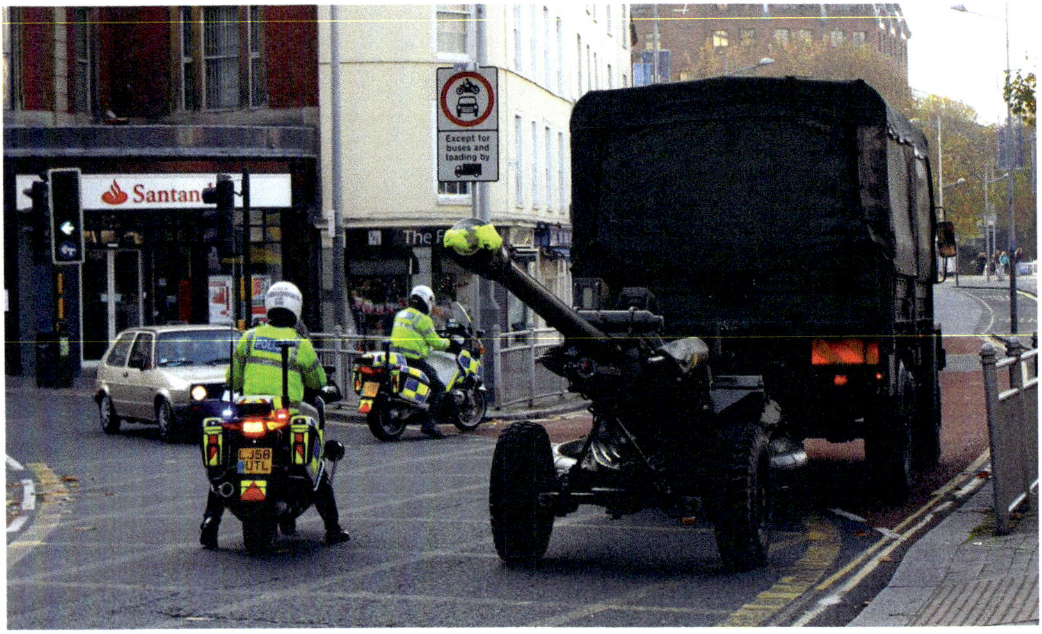

Two military guns are traditionally fired in Bristol to mark the beginning and end of the nation's two-minute silence. Traffic from Baldwin Street is momentarily halted to allow military personnel access to Broad Quay to position the guns in readiness for the 1100 hours public civic service at Bristol's Cenotaph, located at the opposite end of the city centre. Remembrance Sunday 2009.

Station Vans

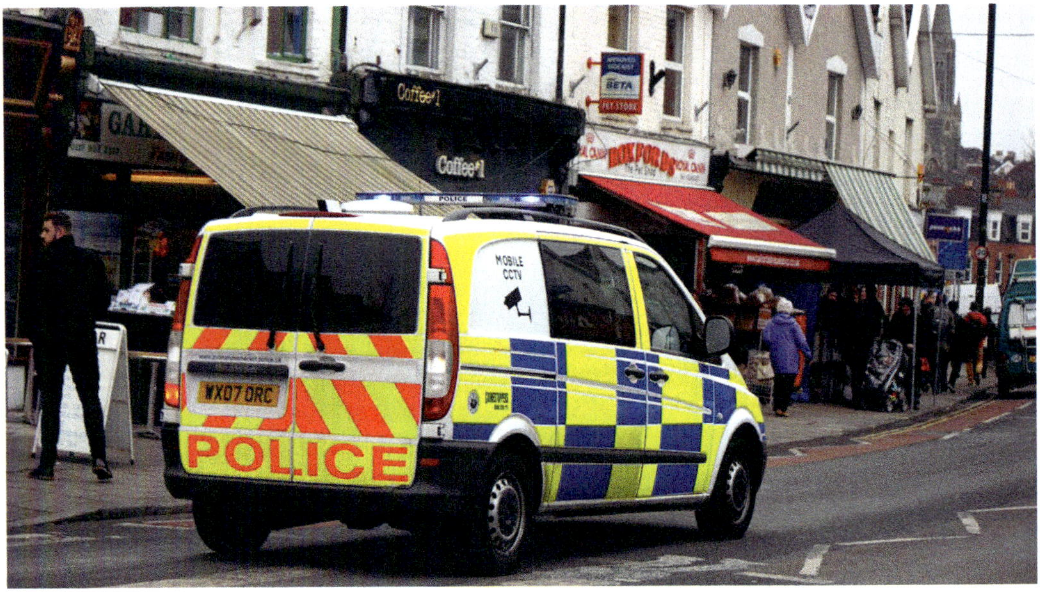

Mercedes Vito cell van WX07 ORC regains speed after slowing for the busy pedestrian crossing by the former Bristol North swimming baths on Gloucester Road, Bishopston, Bristol. 8 February 2015.

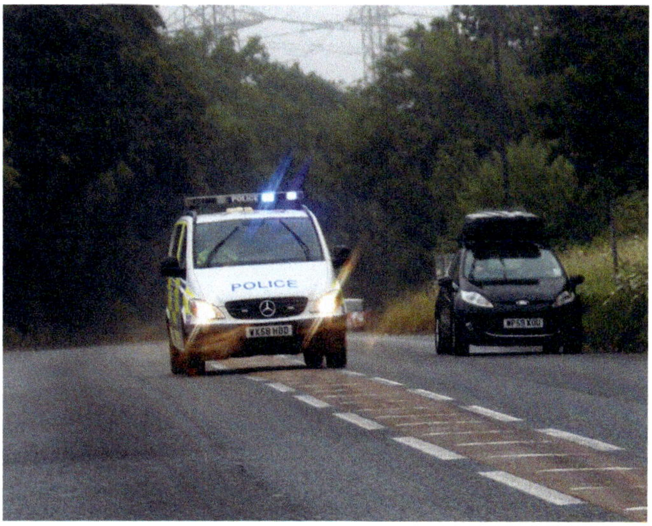

Mercedes Vito van WX58 HDD is captured accelerating hard in the light drizzle as it heads outbound from Yate towards Coalpit Heath on the A432 in South Gloucestershire. 25 July 2016. (Image: Margaret Boulter)

British Transport Police

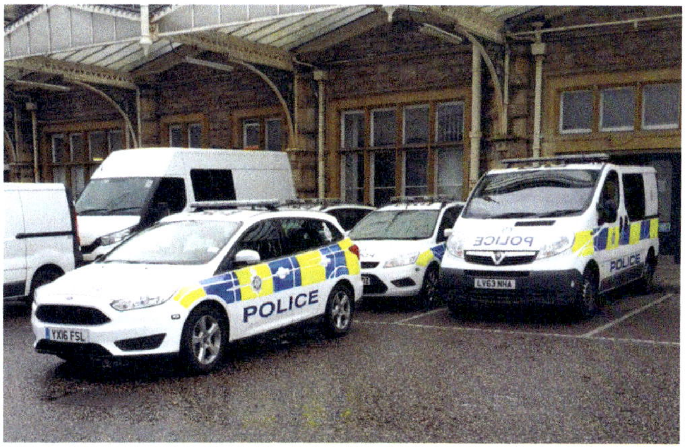

Bristol Temple Meads railway station is a strategic base for British Transport Police (BTP) who cover a considerable radius from this location. In the author's *London Emergency Service Vehicles*, BTP's unique Emergency Response Units feature strongly. 18 November 2016. (Image: Matt Holmes)

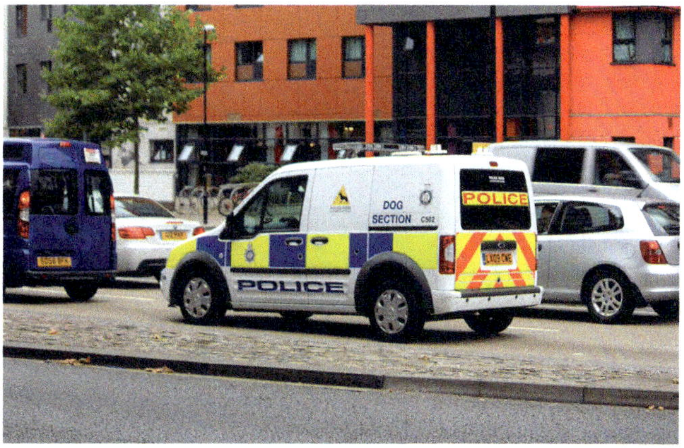

Operating across county boundaries, BTP vehicles and personnel can be seen throughout the region helping safeguard the railways, the travelling public and the vulnerable individuals who, for whatever reason, have strayed near the tracks. 2014.

Conclusion

Air ambulance fundraising and ground support, Dartmoor Rescue Group, Salvation Army, Special Constabulary and Swift Medics – these are just a few other organisations and individuals working in support of the emergency services in the region. Regrettably space constraints do not allow me to do justice to them or all the remaining supporting agencies, many of whom work on a voluntary basis. Nevertheless, a very sincere thank you for what you do.

However, particular mention must be made of control room staff, who in mobilising appropriate resources have the harrowing task of being the first to be contacted by distraught callers using the 999 system. At the opposite end of medically related 999 calls are NHS hospital staffs of all grades who do a fantastic job in accident and emergency departments, in the operating theatres undertaking the most critical of procedures, or providing tender loving care to patients at a time when gentle words of comfort are needed most.

My thanks go to the organisations covered in these pages, their staff past and present, and to Paul Billett, Martin S. Curtis, Professor Adam Dinham, Jamie Enright, Matt Holmes, John Lockwood, Paul Palmer, Navees Rahman, Lee Ralph, James Roberts and Charlotte Stacey. Thanks go especially to my wife Margaret, for her skill with the camera.

Dave Boulter MBE